KETO *for* VEGETARIAN

Cleanse Your Body with The Ultimate Plant-Based Ketogenic Diet for Weight Loss, Burn Fat, Boost Energy, Calm Inflammation and Improve Your Health with 50 Effortless Low Carbs Recipes (with images)

Michelle Simmons

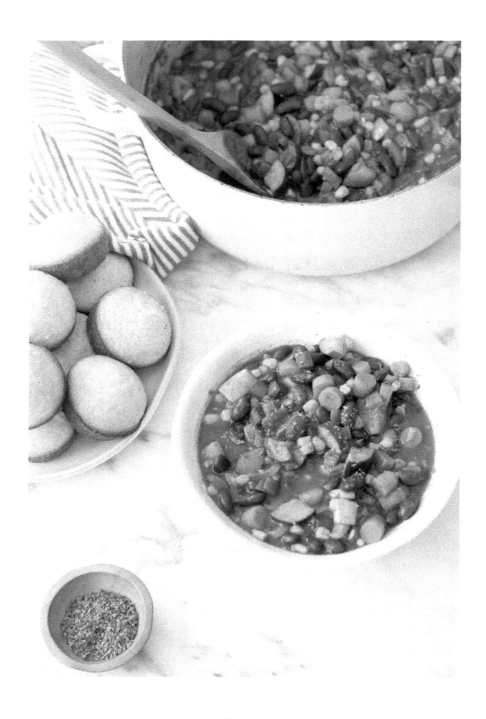

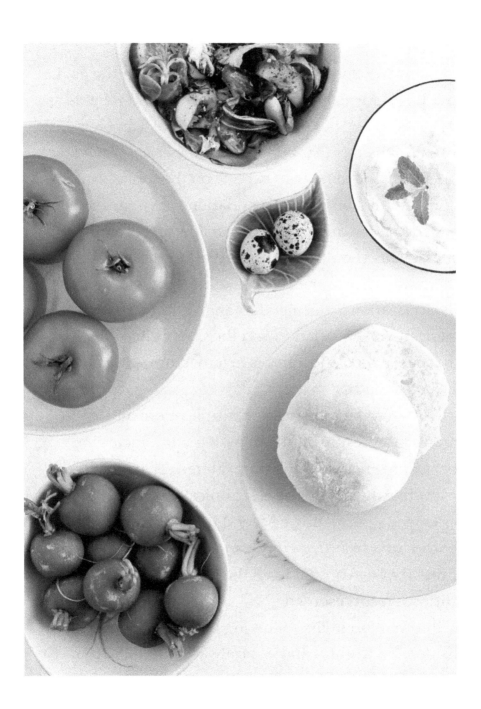

question by the reader will render any resulting actions solely under their purview. There are no scenarios in which the publisher or the original author of this work can be in any fashion deemed liable for any hardship or damages that may befall them after undertaking information described herein.

Additionally, the information in the following pages is intended only for informational purposes and should thus be thought of as universal.

As befitting its nature, it is presented without assurance regarding its prolonged validity or interim quality.

Trademarks that are mentioned are done without written consent and can in no way be considered an endorsement from the trademark holder.

Table of Contents

Introduction

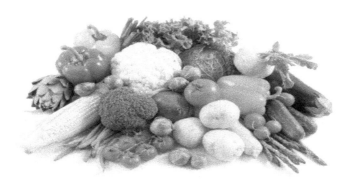

As the main energy source, when carbohydrates are substituted with healthy fats, the body enters a metabolic condition called ketosis. The surplus glucose saved in the body is lost by continuing to eat a high-fat diet. By producing ketones rather than glucose, the body becomes extremely effective at burning fat for use as energy. A ketone is an acidic organic compound that is released when ketosis is present in the blood.

What to do when the Keto flu Hits You!
For much of your energy needs, the keto flu is caused by your body's transition from burning glucose to burning fat. The brain and other organs need some time to adapt to fat rather than sugar for fuel production once ketosis starts.

It is important to consider that many toxins in the body are contained in fat. These accumulated toxins are released into circulation as fat is broken down. The liver must adequately detoxify and remove them from the body to prevent reabsorption of these pollutants.

Those on a keto diet often experience symptoms associated with toxin reabsorption or what is often referred to as the keto flu. The keto flu symptoms typically occur during the first week of a ketogenic diet, especially during the first 3-5 days. The "keto flu" could occur during this period. Fatigue, headaches, irritability, "brain fog," lack of energy, dizziness, cravings for sugar, nausea, and muscle cramps may be signs.

When on the keto diet, if you have these "flu" symptoms, you must hydrate yourself well, maybe even increasing your water and salt consumption. Ensure that you keep a good balance of nutrients, consume more fat, and decrease physical activity until you feel better. By detoxifying yourself before you start the Keto diet, you can also aid your transformation into ketosis and inhibit keto flu symptoms. Find out more, specially built for this, about our Detox Keto Before 6 TM pack.

What does a Ketogenic Diet mean?
In the background of research for epilepsy treatment, the ketogenic diet was born. Trials at John Hopkins Medical Center were performed in the 1920s.

Researchers found major health benefits and even decreased attacks in patients by lowering food consumption for a while or fasting.

Improved heart protection and insulin levels, as well as weight loss, were other noteworthy benefits.

The ketogenic lifestyle, which reproduces these positive results for the body, has been established because fasting is not sustainable in the long term.

The traditional ketogenic diet (or keto diet) consists of a regimen containing high fat, medium protein, and very low carbohydrate intake. The sugars and starches found in foods such as candy, cereals, dairy products, and starchy vegetables are carbohydrates.

Basically, by adopting an LCHF (low-carb, high-fat) regime, the aim is to train the body to use healthier fats instead of carbohydrates for energy. Avocado, cheese, whole eggs, or fatty fish are some examples of good fats.

Most of us would admit that we like consuming carbs, but we dislike the energy drop and the many unwelcome results it sometimes brings. The body retains fat and burns glucose for energy while eating a high-carbohydrate diet. The body enters a ketosis state via the ketogenic diet, which breaks down fats and uses them as an energy source.

Initially, going from a high-sugar diet to a low-carb, high-fat diet (LCHF) may sound like a radical shift since many diets concentrate on sugar, bread, and pasta.

However, when you learn the foods to include and avoid, you will soon realize that the ketogenic lifestyle is completely within your reach.

How long would it take for the Ketogenic state to be reached?

It typically takes up to two weeks for ketogenesis to begin (fat burning). However, in order to help you reach ketosis in a matter of days, certain supplements are formulated. Quicksilver Scientific's Keto Before 6 TM is one such product which actively accelerates the path to ketosis.

Vegetarian Keto

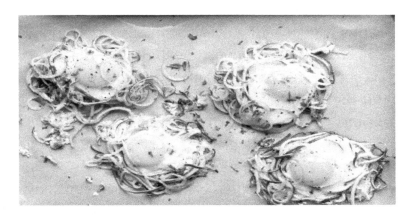

A high-fat, low-carbohydrate, and moderate protein diet, marketed for its strong impact on weight loss and good health, is the ketogenic diet.

There are many animal's origin items on the classic menu of this diet, mainly animal sources of protein.

Given this, a fully vegetarian ketogenic diet can be adopted, only replacing the different animal foods with vegetarian alternatives with proteins and healthy fats.

I will clarify how the diet works in this article and turn it into a cruelty-free diet.

How is it Working?

The ketogenic diet, high in fat and mild in protein, is low in carbohydrates.

To achieve and sustain ketosis, a metabolic mechanism in which the body burns fat for fuel rather than glucose, carbohydrates are usually reduced to less than 50 grams per day.

You lose weight rather than muscle mass due to this diet, giving you a leaner physique.

Moreover, you also lose weight, slimming bloated legs from water accumulation by dramatically limiting carbohydrates. Because this way of eating consists mainly of fat - typically about 75 percent - people consume high-fat animal products such as beef, butter, and fatty dairy products on a ketogenic diet.

It is possible, however, to turn this strictly omnivorous diet into a ketogenic vegan diet.

By depending on high-fat plant products such as coconut oil, avocado, beans, and nuts, vegans will achieve ketosis.

How to Start

Holding the so-called 'macro' (short for macronutrients) under control is one of the keys to a ketogenic lifestyle, i.e., the fats, proteins, and carbohydrates you eat regularly. The total calories contributed by the three groups should be broken down as follows to achieve a state of ketosis: 70-85% fat, 10-20% protein, and 5-10% carbohydrate.

When you start the diet, don't be afraid because it seems like you can't 100 percent respect these proportions. We all lead busy lives, and considering how to integrate the ketogenic diet into your everyday life in a practical way will keep you from leaving in the first few days because you feel like you can't stick to it in the long run.

An adaptation process that requires you to get used to a different lifestyle is important for all new beginnings. And finding the right equilibrium also means making some dietary errors here and there, from which you can learn and get advice for your next ride. In conclusion, don't think too much and concentrate on making the ketogenic diet fun for you.

Variate the Foods
Due to the novelty of eating fatty foods, the transition from a high-carb to a high-fat diet can initially seem enticing. Take the time to find ketogenic diet recipes to avoid tension, allowing you to vary your foods.

When preparing your meals, seeking innovative and simple ideas will help you avoid slipping into monotony.

Don't forget to have plenty of vegetables included. A main source of nutrients in ketogenic diet food plans would be green leafy vegetables. A simple list of foods to include and those to avoid is given below to help you start.

Planning Ahead
The ketogenic diet is doable, but it requires dedication. To make sure you don't go crazy while you're at home or out with friends, prepare your meals in advance. By removing foods that are not adapted to the ketogenic lifestyle, prepare the kitchen. An effective and reliable strategy is to remove anything that may be enticing from the pantry. Replace your junk food stash, candy, and other fast but unhealthy treats with plenty of ketogenic dishes you've prepared. Divide the dishes into smaller portions so that during hunger pangs, they are readily available. You can find that adopting a ketogenic diet can be very difficult while you are out and about. Either way, a little prep is all it takes to overcome this task. To find ketogenic diet alternatives to order next time, search the menus at some of your favorite and famous restaurants.

Efficient Hydration
For any balanced lifestyle, drinking a sufficient amount of water every day is of fundamental importance.
Healthy regular hydration will help you counteract unwanted effects, such as migraines or fatigue, during your ketogenic diet.
It is also necessary for digestion, removing toxins, and appeasing the appetite, generally speaking.

Carrying a bottle of water with you during the day is an excellent way to ensure ample intake.

Once these tips and tricks have been offered to you, all that is left to do is help you prepare your ketogenic meal plan. For ketogenic diets, foods to avoid, and an example of a meal plan for regular meals, read on.

What you should Not eat

You can fully avoid candy and sugar and high-carbohydrate foods such as pasta, rice, bread, flour, and potatoes as a general rule.

Things you Can eat!

Vegetables that rise above the ground and fats that prolong the sense of satiety should be preferred. Green leafy vegetables, crucifers, tomatoes, peppers, peas, celery, eggplants, zucchini and so on are vegetables that rise above the ground.

Keto Vegetarian Recipes

1. Chocolate Termix

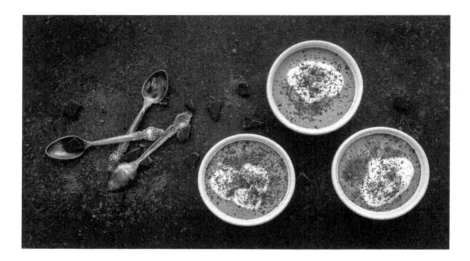

Preparation: 4 hours 20 minutes
Cooking / baking: 10 minutes
Quantity: 5 servings

Ingredients:
- 200 g whipping cream *
- 100 g of dark high percentage chocolate *
- approximately. 50 g sweetener * (honey, coconut sugar, date syrup, erythritol, xylitol, etc. - choose a specific type and amount according to your nutritional style)
- 250 g of fat soft cottage cheese

Method:
1. Heat the cream in a pot almost to a boil.
2. Lower the temperature and let the broken chocolate melt in the hot cream, stirring constantly.
3. You can leave a little chocolate aside for the final decoration (about 10 g is enough for 5 servings).
4. When the chocolate is completely melted, and the mixture is completely smooth, remove it from the plate and stir in the curd.
5. Divide the mass into glasses according to the number of portions and rest in the fridge for at least 4 hours. Upon cooling, the chocolate solidifies again and strengthens the whole mixture.
6. Serve Termix chilled and possibly supplemented with, for example, whipped cream and grated chocolate, the crunchiness will add little fried nuts, and the contrasting acidity will be given by a few teaspoons of forest fruit broth.
7. Termix lasts in the fridge for about 2-3 days. For a little longer storage, leave the termix in one bowl and cover with something.

TIPS:
Instead of whipping cream, you can also use the less fatty one intended for cooking. The resulting termix will be only slightly less dense.
You can mix a little bitter cocoa into the warm cream with melted chocolate and let it dissolve well for a more pronounced taste and color.
Termix can also be used as a filling for various rolls and cuts.
For an interesting color effect, you can layer the chocolate termix into glasses with vanilla and/or fruit termix.
The chocolate for the final decoration is best grated using a vegetable peeler.

---

2. Pumpkin Roll

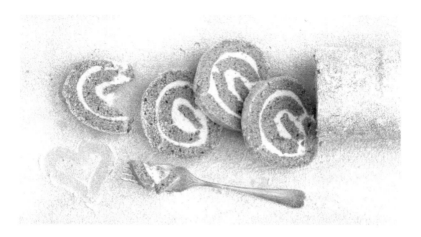

Preparation: 5 hours
Cooking / baking: 40 minutes
Quantity: 6 servings

Ingredients:
1) DOUGH
- 200 g hokaido pumpkin
- 4 eggs
- 80 g almond flour
- 1 teaspoon gingerbread spice or ground cinnamon
- approximately. 30 g sweetener * (honey, coconut sugar, date syrup, erythritol, xylitol, etc. - choose a specific type and amount according to your nutritional style)
- 50 g of pecans or walnuts
- 3 g baking powder (with tartar) or 2 g ordinary

2) CREAM

- 75 g of butter
- approximately. 20 g sweetener * (honey, coconut sugar, date syrup, erythritol, xylitol, etc. - choose a specific type and amount according to your nutritional style)
- a few drops of vanilla extract or grains of 1/2 vanilla bean
- 200 g of creamy cream cheese (e.g., Goldessa or Philadelphia)

Method:
Leave the butter and cream cheese needed for the cream at room temperature at least one hour in advance.

1) DOUGH

1. Remove the seeds from the pumpkin, cut it into cubes, pour it on a baking sheet lined with baking paper, and bake it in an oven preheated to 170 ° C.
2. Bake until soft, approximately 20 minutes. Allow to cool. The weight of the pumpkin should be reduced by about a third by evaporating the moisture.
3. Separate the whites from the yolks.
4. Mix the baked pumpkin until smooth with egg yolks, almond flour, spices, and the chosen sweetener.
5. Mix the crushed pecans or walnuts by hand (they should not be in too large pieces to break the dough, rather than medium-coarse sand).
6. Make the whites into the hard snow and finally whip the baking powder into them.
7. Gently incorporate the protein snow in portions into the pumpkin-nut mixture.
8. Spread the fluffy dough in a layer of about 1 cm on a baking sheet lined with baking paper. Try to create a rectangle with straight sides so that you can make a regular roll better.

9. Place the plate in an oven heated to 170 ° C and bake until golden for approximately 20 minutes.
10. After baking, remove the dough from the oven, place the paper on top of a spread cotton towel, and pull it off.
11. Let the plate exhale for a while and still warm (not hot) along the length with a cloth into a roll. Do not tighten the dough; roll only gently and not tightly.
12. Allow the wrapped to cool completely.

2) CREAM
13. Whisk the permitted butter at room temperature with a mixture of selected sweetener (if it has a coarse texture, grind it gently first) and vanilla extract.
14. Beat the cream cheese as well.

   3)ROLL
15. Carefully unwrap the completely cooled baked plate and spread it with cream. Leave a few inches on the shorter side without filling.
16. Roll the dough with the cream firmly along the length (towards the side without filling) into a roll. Wrap in baking paper and store in the refrigerator for a few hours to solidify the cream and strengthen the roulade.
17. After cooling, cut into slices and serve.

TIPS:
Because the dough lacks gluten, it does not have the flexibility of conventional flour. In part, this property can be "caught up" by adding psyllium or xanthan gum, for example. Personally, however, I would rather have an imperfect roll. That's why you won't find them in the recipe.
To avoid breaking the baked plate as much as possible, try to follow a few steps. Do not bake the dough too much. It should remain pleasantly moist, not completely dry.
But it has to be easy to remove the baking paper. Roll the baked plate into a tea towel while it is still warm.

Just indicate the shape of the roll, do not tighten the dough into the cloth.

Unpack only after it has completely cooled down. This will take a little longer due to tangling, so be patient.

If your dough breaks despite all your efforts, don't despair. Finer cracks will subtly heal after being smeared with cream, so no one will even notice in the final. In the event of a "total disaster," break the dough and fill the glasses with cream layers. Or mix it with the cream, make balls, let cool and wrap in chocolate. You can always pretend it should be

If you do not dare to roll, you can prepare slices. Do not tangle the baked plate. Cut it in half, spread with part of the cream, cover with the other half of the dough, and spread with the rest of the cream. On top, you can make a sprinkle similar to that of carrot slices or pumpkin cashew cashews.

In addition to almond flour, other finely ground nuts or sunflowers can also be used.

You can replace pumpkins with carrots. Just grate it finely before baking.

In addition to cream cheese and butter, you can prepare the filling, for example, from cottage cheese and whipped cream, mascarpone, or even a smooth mix of cashew nuts with a little coconut milk.

If you will gently mix the sweetener into the cream, leave a few grams aside for the final dusting of the roulade.

3. Pumpkin Gnocchi with Blueberry Sauce

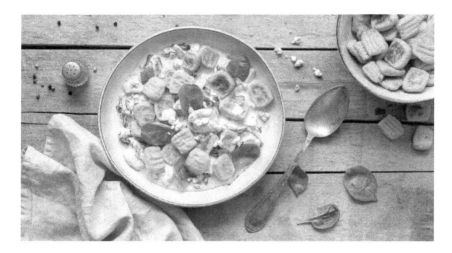

Preparation: 30 minutes
Cooking / baking: 30 minutes
Quantity: 4 servings

Ingredients:
1) NOKY
- 250 g hokaido pumpkin
- 1 egg
- 2 cloves of garlic
- 250 g ricotta
- 60 g of finely grated Parmesan cheese
- 10 g psyllium
- salt

2) SAUCE
- 15 g butter
- 15 g olive oil
- 120 g onion
- 300 g chicken breast or thigh chops
- 200 g whipping cream

- 100 g of blue cheese
- 100 g baby spinach
- pepper

Method:
1) NOKY
1. Get rid of the pumpkin and peel it for the gnocchi's finest possible structure (but this is not necessary for hokaido).
2. Cut the cleaned pumpkin into small cubes, pour on a baking sheet lined with paper, and place in an oven preheated to 180 ° C.
3. Bake until softened pumpkin, approximately 15 minutes.
4. Let the baked pumpkin (its weight should be reduced by about 1/3) cool down and then mix it smoothly with the egg and a little salt (count the salt in Parmesan cheese and sauce, so don't overdo it).
5. Mix the egg mixture with crushed garlic and ricotta. It should not be thin to thicken the dough enough (see TIPS).
6. Finally, mix in the parmesan and psyllium.
7. Work the mixture well and then leave at least Rest for 5 minutes to thicken.
8. Make rolls out of the dough and then cut them into cubes.
9. Gently crush the gnocchi with a fork to create typical strips or gnocchi.
10. Place them on a baking sheet lined with baking paper and bake for approximately 15 minutes at 180 ° C, slightly golden brown.

2) SAUCE
11. Heat the butter and olive oil in a pan and fry the salted onion in a glass.
12. Add the diced chicken meat (for the meatless version, look in the TIPS) and fry gently (be careful not to burn the onions).

---

13. Pour cream into the pan and bring to a boil.
14. Stir in the crushed blue cheese (leave a little to serve if necessary) and cook briefly, constantly stirring, until the cheese is dissolved and the sauce thickens.
15. Back to taste (salt is usually no longer needed, the blue cheese is salty by itself, and a little salt is already in the onion).
16. Remove the pan from the hot plate, add the spinach, cover with a lid and let it dry for a minute.
17. Serve the prepared sauce with baked gnocchi and sprinkle a little crushed blue cheese on a plate.

TIPS:
Ricotta should be as thick as possible and rather drier, so if necessary, let it drip beforehand in a sieve lined with gauze.
I recommend grinding the psyllium finely in a coffee grinder (you can do it together with parmesan cheese).
You can prepare gnocchi in advance. It lasts for about a week in the fridge and for several months in the freezer.
Instead of blue cheese, you can use roquefort or gorgonzola in the sauce; the inside of the brie will also work.
Alternatively, the chicken can be omitted altogether, or mushrooms, for example, can be given instead.

4. "Raffaello" Coconut Balls

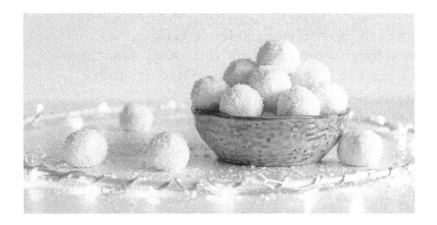

Preparation: 2 hours 30 minutes
Quantity: 30 balls

Ingredients:
- 90 g of coconut butter
- 180 g of red or cream cheese (e.g., Goldessa, Philadelphia)
- 4 tablespoons cream
- approximately. 40 g sweetener * (honey, coconut sugar, date syrup, erythritol, xylitol, etc. - choose a specific type and amount according to your nutritional style)
- 30 g grated coconut
- 30 almonds (preferably blanched)

Method:
1. Gently heat the coconut butter (be careful not to confuse it with coconut oil, that's something else). It must not be overly hot. It can be dissolved at low temperature on a hotplate, in an oven, in a water bath, or at low power in a microwave.

2. Mix the heated (but not hot) coconut butter with the cervix and dilute with cream as needed (add gradually). The mass should be pleasantly soft (it hardens a lot after cooling) but can be shaped in the fingers.
3. Sweeten the mixture to taste. If you use a coarser loose sweetener, I recommend grinding it finely or pre-dissolving it in a little cream.
4. Gradually remove small pieces from the mass, wrap 1 almond in each case, make balls and wrap in grated coconut.
5. Store the balls in the refrigerator, where they solidify after cooling. Keep them covered and use them within about 1 week.
6. Allow them to "exhale" at room temperature for a few minutes before serving, letting go slightly.

5. Tomato Jam

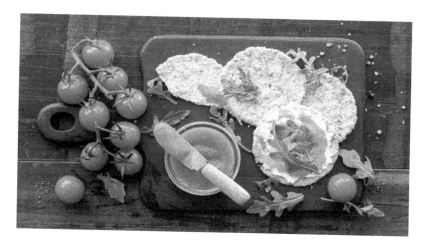

Preparation: 1 hour
Cooking/baking: 45 minutes
Quantity: 20 servings (1 serving = approximately 1 tablespoon)

Ingredients:
- 300 g tomatoes (preferably cherry or date palm)
- 150 g of unpeeled apple
- 50 g sweetener according to dietary style (honey, coconut sugar, date syrup, erythritol, xylitol, etc. - choose a specific type and amount according to your nutritional style)
- 50-100 ml of water
- 50 ml of lemon juice
- a pinch of salt
- grains of 1/2 vanilla bean
- a pinch of chili spice or flakes (optional)

Method:
1. Prepare the jam, choose beautifully ripe tomatoes, preferably cherry or date (they have a more intense taste, a softer skin and are not so floury).
2. Wash the tomatoes and the unpeeled apple and cut into pieces
3. Pour them into a pot, add half of the selected sweetener, pour a little water (as needed) and half of the prepared lemon juice. Add a pinch of salt.
4. Bring to a boil and leave uncovered to bubble gently for approximately half an hour.
5. Stir occasionally and mash the apple pieces.
6. Sift the mixture thoroughly through a fine sieve to get rid of the skins and seeds.
7. Taste the strained jam with vanilla grains and possibly a pinch of chili.
8. Cook to the required density.
9. Taste and add sweetener and lemon juice as needed. Keep in mind that jam is always used only a little, so its taste should be really strong. Also, it cools down a little after cooling.
10. Fill rinsed glasses with boiling water with hot mixture. Close them, turn the lid down and let it cool down. Then store them in the refrigerator, where they last up to several weeks. However, the jam can be consumed almost immediately after cooling.
11. Tomato jam goes well with all cheeses (such as camembert or gorgonzola) or just spread on your favorite crackers. It is also possible to taste meat roast with it.
12. There are sesame crackers, homemade meadows, and arugula in the photo, which will perfectly complement it with its mild bitterness.

6. Spicy Fermented Radish

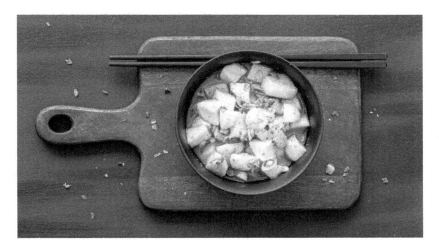

Preparation: 23 hours 55 minutes
Quantity: 10 servings

Ingredients:
- 700 g of radish
- 10 g of sea or Himalayan salt
- 70 g apples
- 20 g of fresh ginger
- 20 g of garlic
- 30 g fish sauce *
- 10 g chili spice (see TIPS)
- 70 g spring or gourmet onions

Method:
1. Peel a radish, wash it and cut it into 1-2 cm cubes.
2. Pour into a sieve, mix and mix gently with salt.
3. Place the sieve on a higher bowl (so that its bottom does not bathe in the drained juice) and, with occasional

stirring, leave the salted radish approximately. An hour to rest.

4. Cut the peeled apple into cubes and ginger into thin slices (cut through the fibers, or grate the ginger).
5. Add crushed garlic, fish sauce, and chili spices. If you don't like spicy foods, reduce the amount of chili used, or omit it altogether, or use traditional Korean chili "gochugaru" (see TIPS).
6. Add dripped radish juice and mix everything until smooth. The mixture should be significantly salty and hot. However, both tastes will be slightly reduced by fermentation, so don't be so afraid of them.
7. Mix the dripped radish (do not rinse it) with the washed chopped delicacy onion and the prepared infusion.
8. Transfer everything to boiling water-washed taller closable jars (we need as little surface area as possible) and stuff as much as possible to remove any air bubbles.
9. The infusion should overlap the radish cubes. If this is not the case, you can load the radish with, for example, a suitable glass that fits under the closed lid and also dilute the infusion with a little salted water.
10. Gently close the glass (do not tighten the lid all the way) and let it stand at room temperature (out of reach of the sun).
11. The glass contents will start to ferment (ferment) after a few hours - bubbles will rise to the surface, and the radish will start to smell pleasantly acidic. How quickly this happens depends very much on the ambient temperature (in winter, it takes longer, in a warm environment faster). Mostly count on12-24 hours.
12. After a few hours of the fermentation process and significant bubble formation, start tasting (always scoop with clean utensils). When the vegetables start to taste the way you like them, you can move the fermented radish to

the fridge. Fermentation will continue in it but will slow down significantly. I like radish the most after about 36 hours at a room temperature of about 22 ° C and at least another 2 days in the refrigerator.

13. Fermented radish lasts stored in the refrigerator for several weeks to months (the longer the time, the more intense the taste).

14. Use it as a spicy supplement to various dishes. Especially for the fatter ones, it will help you with their digestion.

TIPS:
This recipe comes from Korean cuisine and, as with classic kimchi, it traditionally uses Korean chili "gochugaru."
It has a slightly different taste than the one commonly sold (it burns less due to the seeds removed before grinding, it is sweeter and has a pleasant smoky taste.
If you do not have a radish, you can replace it with a kohlrabi-like taste and consistency. However, other vegetables can also be fermented in a similar way (cabbage and Beijing cabbage, carrots, cauliflower, radishes, zucchini).
For fermented Ingredients, the salt used (type and quantity) significantly affects the overall result. If possible, do not use iodized salt, which inhibits the fermentation process. Each salt has a slightly different taste and strength; each vegetable needs a slightly different amount; it also depends on your taste.
Therefore, play with the salt a little while fermenting. However, the more it eats, the crispier and intense the vegetables will be. However, too much salt can spoil the vegetables' taste and slow down the fermentation itself.
With less salt, you will achieve faster fermentation but also less pronounced taste and shorter shelf life.
An adequate amount of salt protects against the formation of unwanted bacteria, but on the contrary, does not prevent the multiplication of the "good" (lactic fermentation).

—

For basic orientation, you can use a tool to help determine the amount of salt used. For every 100 g of Ingredients used (including water), 2 g of salt should come. Do not forget to include the salt in the fish sauce (count on about 3.5 g of salt in 1 tablespoon of fish sauce). For a start, try 1.7 g of salt for every 100 g of Ingredients used. When you taste the fermented vegetables for the first time after a few hours, you can add salt. Just remember the meaning of salt above. So not a little, but not much

If you add water to vegetables, ideally use filtered or boiled and stand to evaporate the chlorine contained. Expect the added water to reduce the concentration of spices and salt used, adding them if necessary.

Adding clean water can be a solution if you find the infusion too salty and spicy. However, its taste changes after fermentation - salinity and spiciness are slightly softened, and, conversely, a pleasant sour taste is added.

Used apple speeds up fermentation, but there is no smell in the resulting taste. Alternatively, you can replace it with the same amount of pear or onion (someone also uses kiwi or pineapple or even Sprite) or cut a little carrot into noodles. For a finer structure of the infusion, you can replace the apple with squeezed apple juice.

When preparing, pay attention to sufficient hygiene - wash all used Ingredients and aids, or use rubber gloves. This will prevent the clogging of unwanted bacteria that could disrupt lactic fermentation and ruin your entire job. Unfortunately, you can find out that this happened by the unpleasant odor or white coating on fermented vegetables' surface.

Do not use a metal container for fermentation.

The glass used for fermentation should be as full as possible to minimize the amount of air between the vegetables and the lid's surface. On the other hand, do not fill it to the brim (ideally a few cm below it) - the juice will form, and the resulting gases could push it out. In this case, support the glass with a tray or plate during fermentation.

Thanks to chili and ginger's action, Korean fermented radish does not tend to catch so-called kris (an undesirable layer of yeast that sometimes forms in fermented vegetables).

If you want to reduce the probability of its occurrence, pay close attention to hygiene, do not use any "started" vegetables and cover the surface of loaded vegetables or cover with a thoroughly washed plastic bag filled with water (the glass does not need to be closed with a lid).

If you plan to ferment vegetables more often, I recommend buying a container designed specifically for fermentation (for example, from Tescom).

If you are not used to fermented vegetables, start consuming them only in small amounts from the beginning (approximately. 1-2 tablespoons a day) and gradually increase them.

Fermented vegetables are a great source of vitamins, enzymes, and also bacteria beneficial to our intestinal microflora.

Therefore, especially in winter and perhaps after taking antibiotics, include it in the diet.

7. Nougat and Chocolate Cupcakes

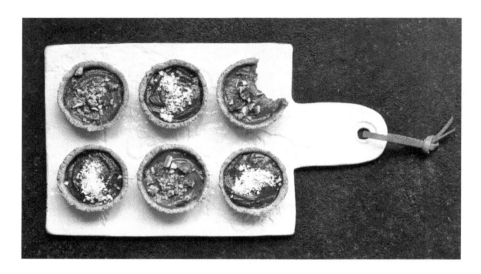

Preparation: 2 hours
Cooking/baking: 45 minutes
Quantity: 6 servings (2 baskets per 1 serving)

Ingredients:
- 175 g of hazelnuts
- 1 egg
- 75 g whipping cream
- approximately. 30 g sweetener (honey, coconut sugar, date syrup, erythritol, xylitol, etc. - choose a specific type and amount according to your nutritional style)
- about 10 g of bitter cocoa
- 120 g mascarpone (at room temperature)
- 45 g of dark high percentage chocolate

Method:

1. Put the hazelnuts in the oven heated to 150 ° C and let them roast for approximately half an hour.
2. Then pour them into a cotton cloth, let them cool for a while and remove them from the skins by rubbing.
3. Crush the cleaned nuts to a fine flour (in an electric coffee grinder or small chopper).
4. Take 100 grams aside and mix them with the egg in a slightly sticky dough.
5. Divide the dough into 12 equal parts (2 parts per serving, approximately 12 g of dough per basket).
6. Use your fingers to form thin cups inside the muffin molds.
7. Put them in an oven heated to 150 ° C and bake for approximately 15 minutes.
8. Then carefully peel them out of the molds and return them upside down to reach the open cooling oven.
9. Grind the second part of the nut flour even finer, except for the nut butter (you can also use the purchased ones). Expect it to take some time. But you need the finest possible structure, so be patient.
10. Mix fine walnut butter smoothly with cream, cocoa, and half a sweetener. Allow to cool.
11. Heat the chocolate to a low temperature in a small pan. Mix it with mascarpone and the other half of the sweetener until smooth. Allow to cool for a while.
12. Fill the baked and cooled cupcakes with the prepared creams - half the amount of nougat and the other half of chocolate, always about 30 g of cream per 1 cupcake.
13. For decoration, you can sprinkle the nougat cupcakes with a little crushed hazelnut, while chocolate cupcakes sprinkle with a pinch of grated cocoa butter.
14. Serve the cupcakes chilled.

8. Ricotta Roll with Sun-Dried Tomatoes

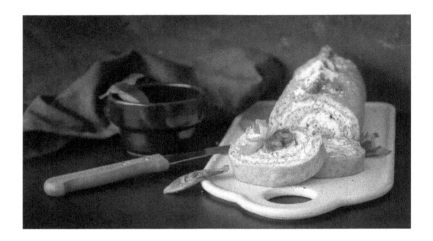

Preparation: 4 hours 30 minutes
Cooking / baking: 20 minutes
Quantity: 4 servings

Ingredients:
1) DOUGH
- 70 g of sunflower seeds
- 200 g of ricotta or cream cheese
- 4 eggs
- 50 g dripped dried tomatoes
- 5 g of baking powder with tartar or 3 g of ordinary
- salt

2) FILLING
- 250 g of ricotta or cream cheese
- 1 large handful of fresh herbs (basil, parsley, etc.)
- 20 g butter
- 2 cloves of garlic
- salt

Method:
1) DOUGH
1. Finely grind sunflower seeds.
2. Mix ground seeds, ricotta, eggs, sun-dried tomatoes, baking powder, and a pinch of salt into a thin fluffy dough.
3. Pour the dough onto a baking sheet lined with baking paper and spread in a pancake less than an inch high.
4. Place in an oven heated to 160 ° C and bake for approximately 20-25 minutes.
5. The pancake should turn golden and strengthen. However, the dough must not dry out too much to roll well.
6. Peel off the baking paper from the warm baked plate, roll the pancake and its length along with it and let it rest for a while.

2) FILLING
7. Mix smooth ricotta, herbs, warmed (not hot) butter, garlic, and salt.
8. Spread the mixture on the baked dough and wrap it tightly in a roll.
9. Save for approximately 4 hours to the fridge.
10. After cooling, cut the roulade into slices and serve as a small snack, breakfast, or supplemented with vegetable salad as a main course.
11. The slices of roulade can also be used as food packed with you on trips.

9. Pumpkin Soup with Sour Cream

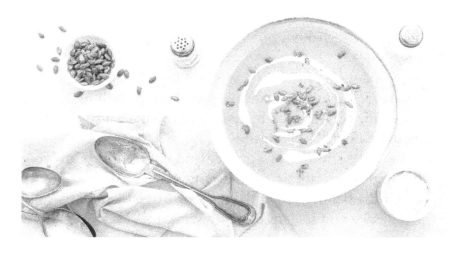

Preparation: 10 minutes
Cooking / baking: 30 minutes
Quantity: 3 servings

Ingredients:
1) PUMPKIN SOUP
- 13 g of ghee or olive oil
- 80 g of onion
- 1 clove of garlic
- 500 g butter pumpkin or hokaido
- 1/2 teaspoon rosemary
- 500 ml of broth or water
- 80 g sour cream
- a little of lemon juice
- salt
- pepper

2) CRISPY SEEDS
- 3 g of ghee or olive oil
- 30 g peeled pumpkin or sunflower seeds
- 1/3 teaspoon rosemary
- a little of lemon peel
- salt

Method:
1) PUMPKIN SOUP
1. Fry the finely chopped onion until golden. Add salt to the juice and fry faster.
2. Add the crushed garlic and let it simmer briefly.
3. Pour diced purged pumpkin into the pot (peel the butter pumpkin, just wash the hokaido).
4. Roast the pumpkin with frequent stirring (approximately 2 minutes).
5. Sprinkle with rosemary and pour broth or water over the contents of the pot.
6. Cook for approximately 15 minutes.
7. Add 50 g of sour cream to the soup and mix everything until smooth.
8. Season with salt, pepper, and a few drops of lemon juice. Just warm up briefly.
9. Top up the soup on a plate with the rest of the sour cream and roasted seeds (see below).

2) CRISPY SEEDS
10. Roast the pumpkin or sunflower seeds crispy at medium temperature with a little fat, stirring constantly.
11. Add a pinch of rosemary and lemon peel. Salt.
12. Add the seeds to the soup only when served so that it does not lose its crunch unnecessarily.
13. You can use the seeds themselves as a small snack or snack for travel.

TIPS:

If you want to achieve the fullest possible taste of the soup, I recommend baking the pumpkin instead of cooking — whether diced or whole (see recipe for pumpkin soup with coconut milk).

Some butter pumpkins have seeds with thinner skin, so you don't have to throw them out when carved out. To check, cut one, and if the skin is really thin and the center is pronounced, boil the seeds for approximately.20 minutes in significantly salted water.

10. Creamy Ice Cream in Walnut Baskets

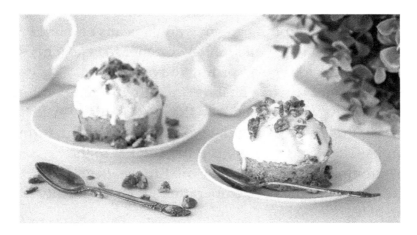

Preparation: 6 hours
Cooking / baking: 25 minutes
Quantity: 6 servings

Ingredients:
1) VANILLA ICECREAM
- 1 vanilla pod or a few drops of vanilla extract
- 250 g whipping cream
- 5 yolks
- 250 g of cottage cheese, mascarpone, yogurt, or cream
- 1 tablespoon vodka or rum (optional)
- approximately. 50 g of sweetener (honey, coconut sugar, date syrup, erythritol, xylitol, etc. - choose a specific type and amount according to your nutritional style)

2)NUT BASKETS
- 100 g of almonds or almond flour
- 1 egg

Method:
1) VANILLA ICECREAM
1. Scrape the grains out of the vanilla pod.
2. In a pot, mix whipping cream, vanilla beans or a little vanilla extract, egg yolks, and sweetener to taste (choose the amount and type according to your habits).
3. With constant stirring, heat the mixture to a temperature of about 85 ° C when it begins to thicken. Caution - watch the temperature well so that the yolks do not boil and form lumps. Therefore, do not keep the hob hot to the maximum. If you feel that the mixture heats up too quickly, lower the hob temperature and occasionally raise the pot.
4. As a result, the cream mixture should have a density like a thinner pudding. A noticeable path should remain on the soaked spoon after wiping with your finger.
5. Allow the cream mixture to cool on the line, stirring occasionally.
6. Mix the curd into the cooled mixture. You can also use mascarpone, yogurt, sour or classic cream. You can play with the variants beautifully and find the best one for yourself.
7. Optionally, a little alcohol can be added, which partially prevents the formation of ice crystals in the hardening ice cream.
8. If you have an ice cream maker at home, use it and follow the instructions. Otherwise, select the following procedure (or the one from TIPS).
9. Pour the mixture into a wider bowl and place in the freezer for approximately 6 hours.
10. Stir the cooling mass from the edges with a fork to break the ice crystals that form, and the resulting ice cream is beautifully soft. From the beginning, once an hour is enough, gradually more often, at the end every 15 minutes.

---

11. After approximately 6 hours, the ice cream should have the correct consistency for serving.
12. If you leave the mixture in the freezer longer and it solidifies completely, let it loosen on the line for a while.

2) NUT BASKETS
13. You can optionally prepare walnut cupcakes for ice cream.
14. Mix finely ground almonds (or other nuts) or almond flour with the egg.
15. Use the finely soaked fingers to create the thinnest possible cups in silicone molds from the stiffer dough.
16. Put them on for 15 minutes in an oven preheated to 150 ° C.
17. Then carefully peel them off, turn them upside down and return to the switched-off cooling oven.
18. Fill the cooled cupcakes with the prepared ice cream and serve.

3) VARIANTS
19. As a variation, you can prepare chocolate ice cream.
20. Heat a little dark chocolate and soak the edges of baked walnut baskets in it.
21. Pour a little hot cream into the bowl with the rest of the melted chocolate, mix and pour the mixture into a pot instead of adding vanilla. Then proceed in the same way as for vanilla ice cream.
22. Another option is fruit ice cream.
23. Optionally omit the vanilla and mix a little mixed fruit into the cooked egg yolk mixture.

11. Mojo Rojo and Mojo Verde Sauces

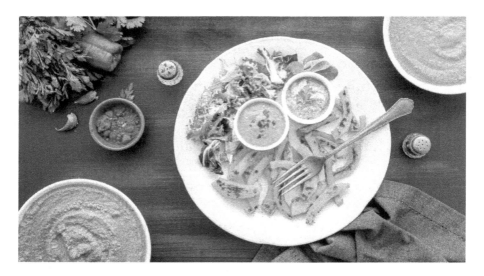

Preparation: 10 minutes
Quantity: 8 servings (from each sauce)

Ingredients:
1) MOJO ROJO SAUCE (RED)
- 400 g fresh red peppers
- 4 cloves garlic
- Ičky teaspoons of chili flakes or chili spices
- 1 teaspoon of ground cumin
- 1 teaspoon smoked or sweet pepper
- 2 tablespoons wine vinegar
- 3 tablespoons olive oil
- 40 g of sunflower seeds
- salt
- pepper

2) MOJO VERDE SAUCE (GREEN)
- 400 g fresh green peppers
- 4 cloves garlic

- 1 teaspoon of ground cumin
- 1 large handful of smooth parsley
- 1 large handful of coriander
- 2 tablespoons wine vinegar
- 3 tablespoons olive oil
- 40 g of sunflower seeds
- salt
- pepper

Method:
1. Clean the pepper and cut it into pieces.
2. Mix it smoothly with all other ingredients.
3. Serve the resulting sauce with roasted vegetables as a fresh dip.
4. But it is also great for roast meat (for example, when grilling) or as a sauce for zucchini noodles.
5. For longer storage, transfer it to glasses, pour olive oil over the surface and store it in the refrigerator.

12. Cauliflower Hummus

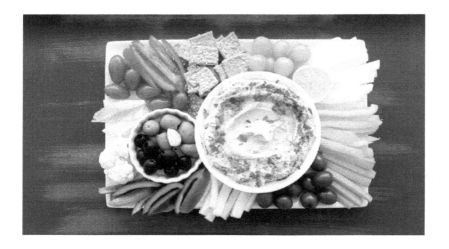

Preparation: 15 minutes
Cooking / baking: 45 minutes
Quantity: 4 servings

Ingredients:
- 600 g of cauliflower
- 60 g carrots or pumpkins or sweet potatoes (optional)
- about 3 tablespoons olive oil
- 2 cloves garlic
- 1/2 lemon
- 50 g tahini
- water as needed
- 1 teaspoon ground cumin
- 1/2 teaspoon smoked, sweet or hot peppers
- salt

Method:
1. Disassemble the cauliflower into small roses.
2. Pour them onto a baking sheet lined with baking paper, add chopped carrots, pumpkin or sweet potatoes (optional, just for taste and color) and mix with a little olive oil.
3. Put the vegetables in an oven heated to 180 ° C and bake for about 45 minutes until the cauliflower softens. Occasionally ruffle the vegetables during baking so that they do not burn.
4. Crush roughly unpeeled garlic by blowing over the knife's surface and pour it over the lemon juice.
5. Let it rest before the vegetables are baked, press it through the press (garlic does not need to be peeled). This crushing method will help the garlic retain its aroma, but its taste was not so pungent.
6. Mix the baked vegetables until smoothly together with the crushed garlic and a few drops of lemon juice.
7. Add tahini (see TIP below), cumin and salt. If necessary, add a little water and mix everything.
8. Make sure that the mixture is as smooth and softly fluffy as possible. Expect it to take a while (depending on the performance of your blender, of course).
9. Continuously taste and add water, lemon, salt, and cumin as needed.
10. Finally, mix in a little olive oil. Count on its bitterness, so give a few drops at the beginning and add later if necessary.
11. Serve cauliflower hummus at room temperature, drizzled with olive oil, sprinkled with cumin, a pinch of smoked, sweet, or hot peppers, and parsley or coriander leaves. Top it up on the table with a pile of fresh vegetables and

---

possibly some favorite crackers, such as flaxseed with parmesan cheese (serving with crackers does not apply to Whole30).

13. Pickled Hermelìn Cheese

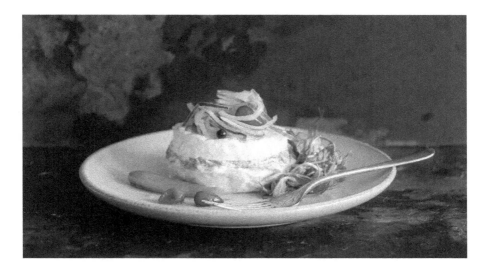

Preparation: 20 hours
Quantity: 3 servings

Ingredients:
- 4 pieces of camembert *
- 2 cloves garlic
- 1 teaspoon barbecue grill
- salt as needed
- 40 g pickled hot peppers (in brine)
- 120 g of onion
- 2 bay leaves
- 5 balls of new spices
- about 250 ml of light olive oil (or quality sunflower) *

Method:
1. Cut one camembert into small cubes, or grate roughly.
2. Mix it with crushed garlic and barbecue spices. If necessary, add salt to taste (depending on the amount of salt in the grill spices).
3. Cut the remaining cheeses into halves. Grease one half of each cheese in the cut with the spiced mixture, cover with the other half, and press together.
4. Gradually stack the prepared cheeses (you can cut them into wedges), hot peppers, thinly sliced onions, and spices in a suitable glass.
5. Fill everything with oil so that the cheese is completely submerged and there are no air bubbles anywhere.
6. Close the container and let it stand at room temperature for 1-2 days. Then store it in the fridge for another few days until the camembert has a beautiful appearance.
7. It is good to let the cheese stand at room temperature for a while before serving and not to serve it directly from the fridge for the best taste.

TIP:
To prevent the cheese from fermenting, keep the tools used and all the ingredients clean during preparation. Wash your hands thoroughly, rinse the glass with boiling water and dry well. Also, make sure that no air bubbles remain in the glass.

14. Baked Bread with Cheese and Tomato Salsa

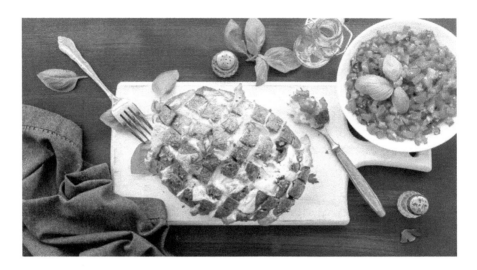

Preparation: 10 minutes
Cooking / baking: 20 minutes
Quantity: 4 servings

Ingredients:
1) BAKED BREAD
- 1 large loaf of yogurt bread
- 2 tablespoons olive oil
- 2 cloves garlic
- 1 small handful of parsley
- salt
- 200 g of hard mozzarella or other hard cheese

2) TOMATO SALSA
- 600 g tomatoes
- 1 handful of fresh basil
- 2 tablespoons olive oil
- 2 teaspoons of wine vinegar

- salt
- pepper

Method:
1) BAKED BREAD
1. To prepare this recipe, use yogurt bread, baked in one large loaf or two (exactly according to the recipe). Of course, other popular pastries can be used.
2. Using a sharp knife, cut the loaf into a grid (see the video recipe). Do not cut to the bottom; the loaf should still stay together.
3. Mix olive oil, crushed garlic, finely chopped parsley, and salt.
4. Using a spoon, apply the mixture to the formed slices in the bread.
5. Cut the mozzarella slices into quarters and the whole cheese into thin wedges. Stuff the cheese evenly into slices in the bread.
6. Place the bread and cheese on a baking sheet and place in an oven heated to 200 ° C.
7. Bake approximately 20 minutes until the cheese melts and turns golden on the surface.

2)TOMATO SALSA
8. Before the bread is baked, prepare the salsa.
9. Cut the washed tomatoes into tiny cubes. Before doing so, remove the watery center with seeds from larger pieces.
10. Put the sliced tomatoes in a sieve, squeeze slightly and let it drip.
11. Mix them with finely chopped basil, olive oil, vinegar, salt, and pepper.

15. Toast Camembert Spread

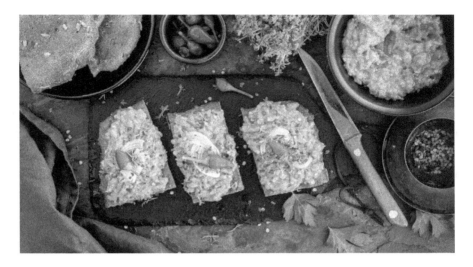

Preparation: 10 minutes
Quantity: 4 servings

Ingredients:
- 240 g of camembert or other blue cheese (camembert, brie, etc.)
- 20 g tomato puree
- 60 g mayonnaise
- 60 g of onion
- 3 cloves garlic
- 10 g pickled hot peppers (in brine)]
- 1 teaspoon sweet pepper
- chili flakes or chili spices to taste
- salt
- pepper

Method:
1. Cut the camembert into small cubes (especially its edges) or grate roughly.
2. Mix it with puree, mayonnaise, finely chopped onion, crushed garlic, and chopped hot peppers.
3. Taste the mixture with sweet peppers, according to the taste of chili, salt, and pepper. You can also add a few drops of hot pepper brine.
4. You can serve the spread immediately, but it tastes best when left in the fridge for at least a few hours.
5. It can be spread on various types of popular pastries, such as seed bread, linen toast, or sesame crackers. An interesting variant is also slice of yogurt bread, which you gently smeared with olive oil and baked sharply in the oven.

16. Baked Mushrooms with Pumpkin Puree

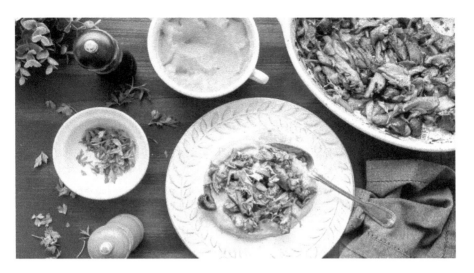

Preparation: 10 minutes
Cooking / baking: 50 minutes
Quantity: 2 servings

Ingredients:
1) ROASTED MUSHROOMS
- 400 g fresh mushrooms (mushrooms, mushrooms, champignons, etc.)
- 60 g shallots
- 50 g bacon or bacon (optional)
- 1 tablespoon olive oil
- 3 cloves garlic
- 1 teaspoon ground cumin
- 1 tablespoon balsamic vinegar
- 1 handful of fresh parsley
- salt
- pepper

2) PUMPKIN MASH
- 500 g butter pumpkin or hokaido
- 1/2 tablespoon olive oil
- 50 g cream cheese (eg Goldessa, Philadelphia)
- salt

Method:
1) ROASTED MUSHROOMS
1. Cut the mushrooms into larger pieces, shallots into wedges and bacon into cubes.
2. Pour the mixture into a baking dish, add salt, pepper and olive oil. Mix everything.
3. Place the uncovered in an oven heated to 180 ° C and bake for approximately half an hour.
4. Add crushed garlic, ground cumin and balsamic vinegar to the baking dish.
5. Mix everything and return to approximately 20 minutes in the oven (along with the pumpkin, see the next part of the recipe).
6. The mushroom mixture's total baking time may vary slightly depending on which mushrooms you use and how high a layer they will lie. If necessary, adjust the time to your liking.

2) PUMPKIN MASH
7. Peel a butter pumpkin; just wash the hokaido.
8. Remove the seeds and cut them into cubes
9. Mix with olive oil and place on 20 minutes in an oven heated to 180 ° C.
10. Mix the baked pumpkin smoothly with cream cheese and salt.

17. Linen Crackers with Parmesan Cheese

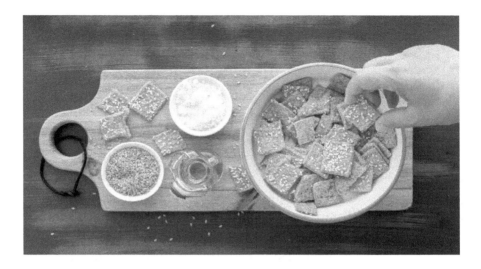

Preparation: 10 minutes
Cooking / baking: 40 minutes
Quantity: 3 servings

Ingredients:
- 40 g of flaxseed
- 40 g finely grated parmesan cheese (parmesan, grana padano, gran moravia, etc.)
- 50 ml of water
- a few drops of olive oil
- 5 g sesame seeds

Method:
1. Grind the flax seeds as finely as possible in an electric coffee grinder.
2. Mix the ground seeds with finely grated Parmesan cheese (Parmesan cheese, grana padano, gran moravia, etc.). If the cheese has a coarser texture, you can grind it along with the flax seeds. The crackers will then be much finer.

3. Add water to the seed-cheese mixture and work everything into a medium-sticky sticky dough. Let it rest for a few minutes.
4. Gently drizzle the restored dough with olive oil (really only a few drops are enough) and roll out the two as thin pancakes as possible between two baking papers. The thinner it is, the more the finished crackers will crunch.
5. Carefully remove the top baking paper from the pancake and sprinkle it with sesame seeds (it can be omitted or replaced with other small seeds - poppy, flax, etc.).
6. Cut the dough into the required shapes and place in an oven heated to 160 ° C.
7. Bake approximately half an hour. Then break the crackers according to the cuts and turn on the plate.
8. Return the crackers about 10 minutes in the oven until beautifully crispy and crispy. Take good care of them in the last minutes, they are easily burned and bitter thanks to the cheese.
9. Serve the finished crackers alone as a small snack, or add them with a favorite spread.
10. They can be stored dry in a closed container. For later serving, I recommend briefly warming them in the oven to restore crispness.

18. Cashew Cakes with Cream Filling

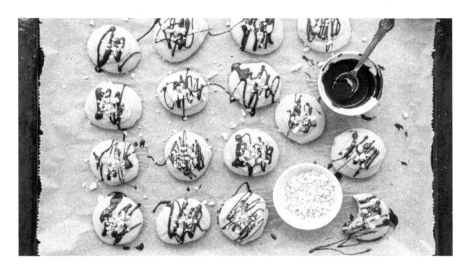

Preparation: 30 minutes
Cooking / baking: 15 minutes
Quantity: 5 servings (1 serving = approximately. 3 cakes)

Ingredients:
- 125 + 15 g cashew nuts
- 5 g of baking powder with tartar or 3 g of ordinary
- 1 egg
- 1 protein
- 1 egg yolk
- 140 g of cream
- 1 teaspoon vanilla extract
- approximately. 10 g sweetener (honey, coconut sugar, date syrup, erythritol, xylitol, etc. - choose a specific type and amount according to your nutritional style)
- 20 g of dark high percentage chocolate

Method:

1. Grind as much as possible finely 125 g of cashew nuts.
2. Mix them with baking powder, 1 egg, and 1 egg white. Work into a smooth dough.
3. Using a spoon, make small buns on a baking sheet lined with baking paper.
4. Then create dimples in each of them using the bottom of a lightly soaked spoon or fingertip.
5. Put the cakes in an oven heated to 150 ° C and bake for approximately 15 minutes. Then allow to cool.
6. Bring the cream to a boil in a smaller pan. While stirring, allow to thicken and boil to less than half its original volume.
7. Stir the vanilla extract into the thick mixture. Turn off the hob to stop boiling.
8. Stir a few teaspoons of hot thick cream into 1 egg yolk and then pour back into the pan, stirring constantly. Caution - the mixture must no longer be boiled.
9. Taste and, if necessary, slightly sweeten.
10. Allow the mixture to cool on the kitchen counter with occasional mixing.
11. Fill the baked cakes with a thick cream mixture and put them in the freezer for a few minutes or in the fridge for at least half an hour.
12. Sprinkle the cooled cakes with melted chocolate and sprinkle with 15 g of coarsely crushed cashew nuts.

19. Pumpkin Cashew Cream Puff with Cinnamon

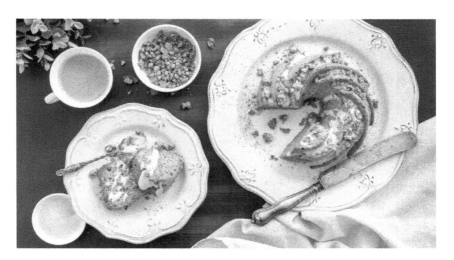

Preparation: 1 hour
Cooking/baking: 1 hour
Quantity: 6 servings

Ingredients:
1) CAKE
- 180 g unroasted cashew nuts
- 150 g hokaido or butter pumpkin
- 3 egg yolks
- 1-2 teaspoons ground cinnamon
- 1/3 teaspoon ground cloves
- a pinch of grated nutmeg
- sweetener (honey, coconut sugar, date syrup, erythritol, xylitol, etc. - choose a specific type and amount according to your nutritional style)
- 3 proteins
- 3 g of baking powder with tartar or 2 g of ordinary

2) POSYPKA
- 40 g cashews
- 1 protein
- 1/2 teaspoon ground cinnamon

3) GLAZE
- 40 g of unroasted cashews
- 10 g butter or ghee
- 80 g of cream or walnut milk

Method:
1) CAKE
1. Finely grind (see note below the recipe) cashew nuts, including those for the icing, and then pour the required amount aside. For the cake's soft structure, it is necessary that the resulting flour is really fine, without larger pieces.
2. Mix the diced raw pumpkin (hokaido just wash, peel the butter), egg yolks, ground cinnamon, cloves, nutmeg, and the chosen sweetener to taste.
3. Mix ground cashew nuts into the pumpkin mixture and work into a smooth, thinner dough.
4. Whisk solid snow from 3 whites. When it starts to harden, add baking powder and work carefully.
5. Gently stir the snow into the cashew dough in portions.
6. Pour the fluffy dough into a cake pan. If you use anything other than silicone, I recommend wiping it thoroughly with butter and sprinkling it with finely ground nuts.
7. Expect the dough to rise in the mold, so it should reach a few centimeters below the edge.
8. If you have dough left or are afraid of tipping the cake out of the mold, you can pour it into smaller molds or simply use a cake tin or a plate lined with baking paper.
9. Place the prepared dough in an oven preheated to 160 ° C and bake according to the mold's size. The dough poured

on the sheet is approximately 20 minutes, in muffins approximately 30 minutes, in a wider cake form approximately 45 minutes, and a small cake will need approximately60 minutes. Do not open the oven during baking so that the dough does not fall unnecessarily.

10. At the end, test the baking of the dough by sticking a skewer. If you remove it completely dry after a few seconds, you can switch off the oven. Otherwise, bake for a few more minutes.

11. For cake and a higher cake body, I recommend leaving the mold with the dough. Walk for 10 minutes in the oven with the door ajar.

12. When using a silicone mold, allow the dough to cool before rolling out. On the other hand, other molds turn the cake still warm a few minutes after removing it from the oven.

2)POSYPKA

13. Crush 40 g of cashew nuts into pieces. They can be broken in a bag and broken with a meat mallet or simply broken in your fingers.

14. Mix them with protein and cinnamon and spread the mixture on baking paper.

15. Put them in an oven heated to 160 ° C. After a few minutes, break the baked mixture into small pieces and return to the oven until the nuts rustle to the touch and bake crisp beautifully. It takes a total of approximately 20 minutes.

3) GLAZE

16. Mix 40 g of pre-ground cashews, which you have set aside, together with butter or ghee even more finely, until a thick cream.

17. Unfortunately, with a smaller number of nuts, the problem is that most mixers are too large and do not process such a small amount. Although the grinder is not designed for

this (!), I use it to prepare a small amount of nut butter. All you have to do is wipe it from the inside with a damp cloth as soon as possible after use.

18. Of course, you can skip this step and use the purchased cashew butter on the icing, or omit the icing altogether.
19. Mix walnut butter with cream (or some walnut milk) to create a thick but partially liquid cream. Keep it at room temperature; it would get too stiff in the fridge.

4) ADMINISTRATION
20. Pour icing over the cooled cake and gently dust it with cinnamon. Sprinkle it with crispy nuts just before serving.

20. Pumpkin Salad with Herbs

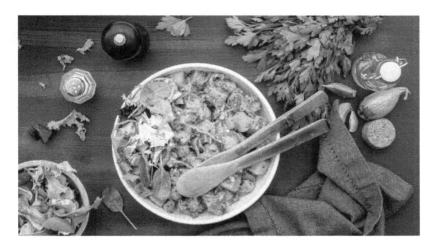

Preparation: 10 minutes
Cooking / baking: 20 minutes
Quantity: 3 servings

Ingredients:
- 750 g butter pumpkin or hokaido
- 2 cloves garlic
- 4 tablespoons olive oil
- 1 large handful of popular fresh herbs (parsley, chives, coriander, basil, etc.)
- 1 tablespoon wine or apple cider vinegar
- 40 g dripped dried tomatoes
- chili (optional and to taste)
- 60 g shallots
- salt
- pepper

Method:

1. Peel a butter pumpkin; just wash the hokaido. Remove any seeds from the pumpkin and cut them into cubes.
2. Mix them with a little olive oil and spread on a baking sheet lined with baking paper. Add unpeeled garlic cloves.
3. Place in an oven heated to 200-210 ° C and bake for approximately 20 minutes.
4. Mix your favorite fresh herbs, olive oil, vinegar, and sun-dried tomatoes into a coarse paste. If you like a spicier taste, you can also add a little chili (whether fresh chili pepper without seeds, flakes, or spices).
5. Cut the peeled shallots into thin strips.
6. Remove the baked pumpkin and garlic from the oven. Squeeze the cloves, spread the soft inside and mix into the prepared herb paste.
7. In a bowl, mix the hot baked pumpkin, herb dressing, and chopped shallots.
8. Add salt and pepper to taste.
9. You can serve the salad immediately. It tastes great, not only warm but also cold. It goes well with roasted or grilled meat.

21. Romesco Sauce

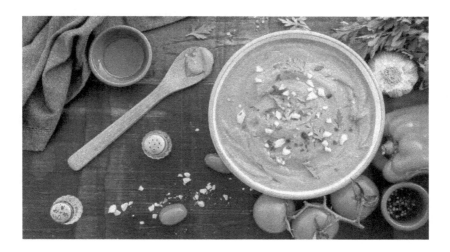

Preparation: 20 minutes
Cooking / baking: 40 minutes
Quantity: 10 servings

Ingredients:
- 800 g fresh red peppers
- 400 g of tomatoes
- 10 cloves of garlic
- 1 chili pepper (optional)
- 4 tablespoons olive oil
- 100 g peeled almonds
- 2 tablespoons wine vinegar
- 1 teaspoon smoked peppers
- salt
- pepper

Method:
1. Place whole peppers on a baking sheet or in a baking dish.
2. Pour the tomatoes into a separate baking dish (cut the larger pieces in half) and gently pour olive oil over them.
3. Add 4 unpeeled cloves of garlic and chili pepper (optional).
4. Put the vegetables in an oven heated to the maximum.
5. Bake approximately 40 minutes (the exact time depends a lot on the size of the peppers and tomatoes and also the power of your oven) until the peppers have black skin.
6. Don't be afraid of a black burnt surface. You will later peel the peppers' skin, and the flesh under it will have a beautiful smoky taste, which makes romesco sauce so good.
7. During baking, turn the peppers at least once to roast them on all sides and mix the tomatoes.
8. While the vegetables are being baked, fry the almonds at medium temperature in a frying pan. Almonds can be whole or chopped but always peeled (the skins would unnecessarily add bitterness to the resulting sauce).
9. Transfer the baked peppers to a bowl and cover. They evaporate, and their toasted skin will peel off better.
10. Squeeze the baked garlic from the skin. Get rid of the chili pepper with the stems and possibly also the seeds if you do not like too spicy food.
11. After a few minutes, take the steamed peppers out of the bowl and remove them from the stems and kernels. Peel the flesh.
12. Mix topped peeled peppers, baked tomatoes and chilies, squeezed baked garlic, peeled fresh garlic, roasted almonds, olive oil, wine vinegar, and smoked peppers.
13. Season with salt and pepper or a pinch of chili flakes.
14. The sauce tastes best the next day when all tastes are beautifully combined. You can serve it hot or cold. It goes

well with baked vegetables, grilled meat, fish, or shrimp. You can dip homemade pastries, popular crackers, or cheese chips (does not apply to Whole30).

15. Store the sauce in the refrigerator, where it will last for several days to weeks.

22. Asparagus Soup with Parmesan Crackers

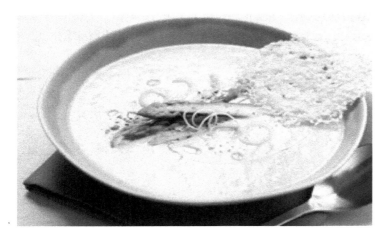

Preparation: 10 minutes
Cooking/baking: 30 minutes
Quantity: 3 servings

Ingredients:
1) KREKRY
- 50 g grated Parmesan cheese
- 50 g almond flour
- 1 protein

2) SOUP
- 500 g of green asparagus
- 30 g butter
- 150 g spring onions (including green part)
- 2 cloves garlic
- 800 ml of water
- 50 g grated Parmesan cheese
- 1 egg yolk
- 50 g of cream
- salt and pepper

Method:

1) KREKRY

1. Mix grated parmesan cheese with almond flour and protein, depending on your taste, salt, and pepper a little.
2. Make a harder dough on a baking sheet lined with baking paper on a thin pancake (the thinner it is, the more it will crunch). For easier work with the dough, soak your fingers in water or smear with olive oil.
3. Cut the pancake into the desired shapes and bake for 30 minutes in an oven heated to 160 ° C. About 10 minutes before the end of the pancake, break according to the cuts and turn the pieces.

2) SOUP

4. Wash the asparagus and get rid of the woody ends (I break it, where it breaks, usually comes exactly to the end of the woody part).
5. Fry the chopped spring onion briefly on the butter at a lower temperature.
6. Add garlic and asparagus. Leave them to roast with occasional shaking5-10 minutes.
7. Cut the tips out of the roasted asparagus and set them aside. Pour water over the pot, salt, pepper, and bring to a boil.
8. Sprinkle with parmesan cheese and mix everything smoothly. Cook briefly.
9. Remove the pot from the hotplate and pour the egg yolk mixed with cream and 2 tablespoons of hot soup into the hot soup. Mix for a short time, but don't cook anymore.
10. Serve the soup garnished with roasted asparagus tips and some spring shoots, complemented by parmesan crackers.

23. Turmeric Calimero

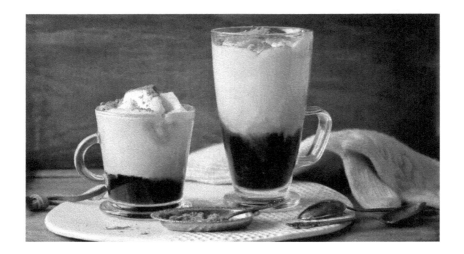

Preparation: 10 minutes
Cooking / baking: 10 minutes
Quantity: 5 cups

Ingredients:
- 250 ml whipping cream
- pinch of ground turmeric
- 3 egg yolks
- grains of 1/2 vanilla bean or a few drops of extract
- 20 g sweetener (honey, coconut sugar, date syrup, erythritol, xylitol, etc. - choose a specific type and amount according to your nutritional style)
- 50 - 100 ml of rum or cognac, or whiskey
- 5 cups of espresso
- a little bitter cocoa

Method:

1. Mix 150 ml of cream with a pinch of turmeric, egg yolks (strain through a sieve to get rid of the white loop), vanilla, and any sweetener.
2. With constant stirring, bring the mixture to a temperature of 80 ° C on a moderately melted plate, where it begins to thicken as a thinner pudding. You must not exceed this temperature to prevent the liqueur from coagulating. Then mix the alcohol to taste (you can omit it or give it more).
3. Make coffee in cups and pour the prepared warm liqueur over it over a spoon (so that the liquids do not combine).
4. Garnish the drink on top with whipped cream from the rest of the cream and lightly dust with bitter cocoa.
5. Drink hot and thoughtfully

24. Linen Toast

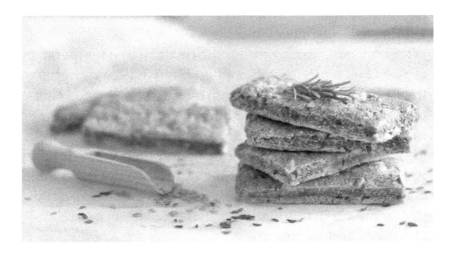

Preparation: 5 minutes
Cooking / baking: 40 minutes
Quantity: 4 servings

Ingredients:
- 60 g finely ground flax seeds or flax flour
- 60 g of coconut flour
- 20 g psyllium
- 40 g peeled sunflower seeds
- 10 g of baking powder with tartar or 6 g of ordinary
- 2 eggs
- 25 g of olive oil
- 200 ml of water
- crushed cumin
- salt

Method:
1. Mix all the ingredients and knead into a medium-hard dough.
2. Taste it according to your choice, for example, with crushed garlic, herbs, or your favorite spice instead of cumin.
3. Make the dough on a baking sheet lined with baking paper on a pancake a few millimeters high, cut it into the required shapes and bake for 30 minutes in an oven heated to 180 ° C.
4. Then separate the toasts to bake them better and put them back in the oven 5-10 minutes.
5. The finished toasts are great for various spreads, steak tartare, or as a base for a snack on the trip.

25. Pumpkin Cream "Rice" with Cinnamon

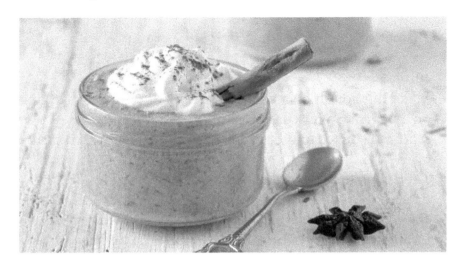

Preparation: 2 hours
Cooking / baking: 25 minutes
Quantity: 3 servings

Ingredients:
- 250 g hokkaido pumpkin
- 150 g + 50 g whipping cream or coconut milk
- 50 ml of water
- 2 stars star anise
- 1 teaspoon ground cinnamon
- a pinch of dried ginger
- 20 g sweetener (honey, coconut sugar, date syrup, erythritol, xylitol, etc. - choose a specific type and amount according to your nutritional style)
- 1 egg yolk

Method:
1. Wash the pumpkin, remove the soft center with seeds, cut into cubes and crush in a chopper or robot into rice-sized grains. Do not use an immersion mixer; you will get porridge (even if it will be good).
2. In a pot, mix pumpkin rice, 150 g of cream or coconut milk, water, spices, and any sweetener (adjust the amount to your liking).
3. Bring to a boil, bring the temperature to a minimum and cover the pot with a lid.
4. Let it gently bubble for around 15 minutes.
5. Then uncover the lid and Slightly raise the temperature for 5 minutes to evaporate excess liquid.
6. Stir the yolk in a small bowl (ideally remove the loops with protein). Add a tablespoon of hot mixture from the pot and stir.
7. Remove the pot of creamy pumpkin rice from the hotplate and add the egg yolk mixture while stirring constantly. It thickens the rice to a pudding consistency.
8. Allow to cool.
9. Fill the glasses with chilled pumpkin rice (remove star anise), garnish with a spoon whipped cream from the rest of the cream or coconut milk, and lightly dust with cinnamon.

PS: If you don't like cinnamon or want to try other flavors, vanilla, cocoa, or a little melted dark chocolate will also work great.

26. Mega Fast Chia Pudding

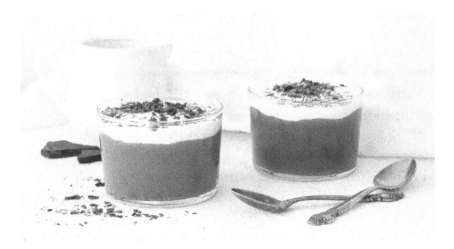

Preparation: 5 minutes
Quantity: 2 servings

Ingredients:
- 25 g of chia seeds
- 200 ml of coconut milk or classic cream for whipping or cooking
- 20 g of bitter cocoa
- 15 g sweetener according to your diet (honey, dates, date syrup, xylitol, erythritol, etc.) *

Method:
1. Grind the chia seeds in an electric coffee grinder as finely as possible.
2. Mix the crushed chia with chilled coconut milk or cream, cocoa, and sweetener.
3. You can serve immediately. Decorate the pudding with a scoop of whipped cream and grated dark chocolate, for example.

27. Pumpkin Brownie Cake

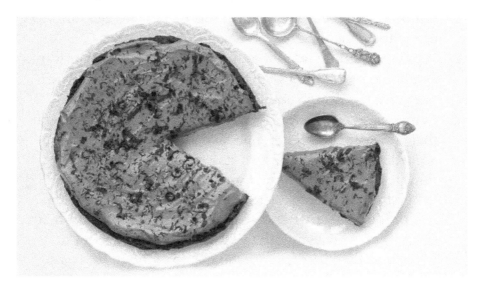

Preparation: 1 hour 30 minutes
Cooking/baking: 25 minutes
Quantity: 6 servings

Ingredients:
- 240 g hokkaido pumpkin
- 2 eggs
- 15 g of coconut flour
- 50 g almond flour
- 10 g of bitter cocoa
- approximately. 40 g sweetener (honey, coconut sugar, date syrup, erythritol, xylitol, etc. - choose a specific type and amount according to your nutritional style)
- 60 g of dark high-percentage chocolate + a few extra grams for sprinkling
- 100 g whipping cream or coconut milk
- 250 g mascarpone (optional)

Method:

1. Finely grate the pumpkin. Mix it with eggs, coconut and almond flour, cocoa, 25 g of the chosen sweetener, and 25 g of melted chocolate.

2. Work everything into a medium-liquid dough. Pour it into a suitable mold lined with crumpled baking paper. For 6 portions, the dough comes out in a cake form with a diameter of 23 cm, approximately 1-2 cm in height. If you make the carcass higher, increase the baking time accordingly. At the dough's stated height, it starts at 25 minutes at 180 ° C. Allow the finished body to cool.

3. While the cake is baking, prepare the icing. Dissolve the rest of the sweetener and chocolate in the cream and mix everything into a smooth mixture. Allow to cool for a while and then incorporate the mascarpone in portions (see note below).

4. Coat the cooled carcass with chocolate mascarpone and sprinkle with grated chocolate.

5. Allow to cool in the refrigerator for at least an hour and then serve sliced.

6. The result is a typically dense, moist brownie. Therefore, if you do not want to do with cream or use dairy products, it is enough to dissolve chocolate and sweetener in cream or coconut milk, and thus drip brownies.

28. Cocoa Pancakes

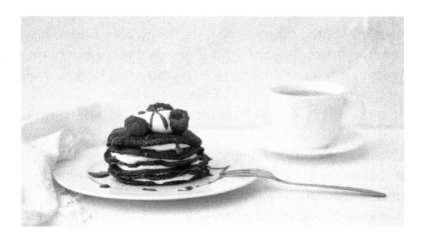

Preparation: 15 minutes
Cooking / baking: 20 minutes
Quantity: 4 servings

Ingredients:
1) PANCAKES
- 40 g of flaxseed or flaxseed flour
- 40 g grated coconut
- 40 g of bitter cocoa (adjust the exact amount to taste)
- 4 eggs L
- 80 g whipping cream
- 60 g sweetener (honey, coconut sugar, date syrup, erythritol, xylitol, etc. - choose a specific type and amount according to your nutritional style)
- ghee for frying

2) GLAZE
- 20 g of dark high percentage chocolate
- 60 g whipping cream
- 200 g creme fraiche, fatty sour cream, or mascarpone

Method:
1. First, grind the flax and coconut finely in an electric coffee grinder.
2. Then mix both smoothly together with cocoa (give less from the beginning and add if necessary), eggs, cream, and sweetener (adjust the amount to your taste here as well).
3. Let the dough stand for a while to thicken.
4. Heat the ghee to a medium temperature in a pan and fry small pancakes on both sides. Approximately 1-2 tablespoons of dough come out for one.
5. Pancakes are very fragile, so turn them only when they solidify from the top.
6. Lubricate the finished pancakes with creme fraiche and pour chocolate melted in hot cream.
7. You can add a few pieces of some berries.
8. If you want to save work and reduce the fat content, bake the oven's pancakes.

29. Cauliflower Porridge

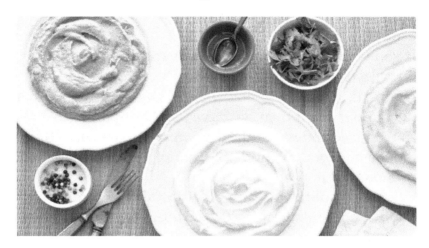

Preparation: 10 minutes
Cooking / baking: 20 minutes
Quantity: 2 servings

Ingredients:
1) BASIC RECIPE
- 550 g of cauliflower
- salt
- pepper

2) VARIANTS
- 160 g carrots, pumpkins, or sweet potatoes
- 30 g butter * or ghee
- 40 g whipping cream *
- 25 g cashews
- 50 g of cream cheese* (Philadelphia, Goldessa, Lučina, etc.)
- 80 g of fresh spinach
- 4 g of garlic

Method:

1. First, remove the cauliflower from the broom, break it into roses and then boil them gently in salted water. Cauliflower should crumble.
2. If you want to prepare an orange variant of porridge, let the selected vegetables cook with the cauliflower.
3. Drain the cooked cauliflower and squeeze through a sieve or cotton cloth. It does not have to be completely dry, such as with croquettes, but the less water remains in it, the more cream you can add, for example, and it will be more pronounced in taste.
4. Squeezed cauliflower (and possibly other vegetables), salt, pepper, and mix until smooth. Continue with one of the options below.
5. For the basic version, it is enough to add ghee or butter to the cauliflower.
6. You can prepare a more classic porridge using cream.
7. An amazing option is to mix cauliflower with cream cheese.
8. For those who avoid dairy products, there is also a variant with cashew nuts. It may sound crazy, but it works great. All you have to do is soak the nuts in lukewarm water at least 2 hours in advance, then melt them and mix them carefully with cauliflower into a perfectly smooth porridge.
9. You can also mix spinach, which you let fade in a pan, where you briefly fried crushed garlic on a small amount of fat, into a white porridge (whether with butter, cream, cheese, or cashew nuts).
10. For effect, you can prepare 2 colors of porridge and then mix them slightly on a late in a circular motion.

30. Cheese Balls

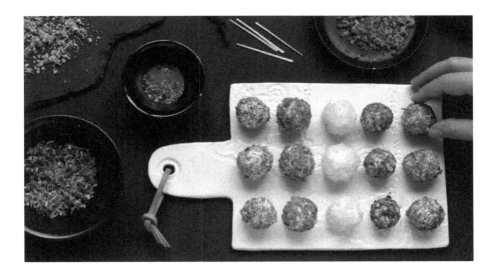

Preparation: 20 minutes
Cooking / baking: 10 minutes
Quantity: 25 balls

Ingredients:
- 200 g cream cheese (Philadelphia, Goldessa, etc.)
- 200 g grated hard cheese (e.g., Gouda, Cheddar, Emmental)
- 20 g nuts (pecans, walnuts, handles, etc.)
- 50 g dried ham (Prosciutto, Parma, Jamon Serrano, etc.)
- 50 g yellow peppers
- 2 g sweet peppers and a pinch of chili
- 2 handfuls of fresh herbs (e.g., parsley, chives, basil)

Method:

1. Drain the excess liquid from the cream cheese. Mix it with grated cheese and let the mass cool in the fridge.
2. Crush the nuts finely (they are best broken in a mortar because they quickly turn into a past in a coffee grinder, the mixer is too big for the stated amount).
3. Cut the dried ham into small cubes and bake them 10 minutes in an oven heated to 180 ° C until they start to rustle to the touch. Dig them occasionally. After removing the ham from the oven, dry it with a paper towel to remove excess grease and let it cool down.
4. Cut the pepper into tiny cubes. Carefully wipe off excess moisture with a paper towel.
5. Mix sweet peppers with chili flakes in a small bowl.
6. Chop the herbs as finely as possible.
7. The cooled cheese mixture makes 25 balls (approximately 15 g per one) and wrap them in 5 pieces in each prepared ingredient.
8. Serve chilled.

31. Unbaked Tricolour Cheesecake

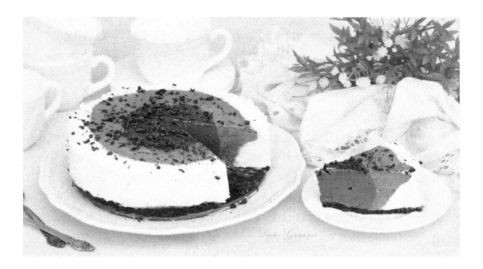

Preparation: 4 hours 20 minutes
Cooking / baking: 5 minutes
Quantity: 8 servings

Ingredients:
- 150 g of pecans or other popular nuts
- 50 g + 40 g + 60 g of dark high percentage chocolate
- (total 150 g)
- 10 g of flavored gelatin *
- 400 ml whipping cream
- 400 g of cream cheese (Philadelphia, Goldessa, etc.) **
- 60 g of sweetener according to your eating style (honey, dates, date syrup, xylitol, erythritol, etc.) - the exact amount depends on the chosen type and your taste
- vanilla extract or granules of 1 vanilla bean

Method:
1. Crush the nuts finely in a blender.
2. In a small skillet, melt the chocolate on a hot plate. Take one-third (the first part of the stated weight) and mix it carefully with walnut pulp (walnut flour can also be used if necessary).
3. Stuff the mass on the bottom of the cake tin (approximately. 20 cm in diameter for 6-8 portions), which you lined with baking paper. Before putting it in the mold, crumple it, soak it in water and squeeze it out of the excess liquid. You will then be able to work with him better.
4. Let the base of the cake cool in the fridge.
5. If you use sliced gelatin, soak it in cold water for a few minutes. Then squeeze it.
6. Heat the cream on a hot plate. Add vanilla to it and dissolve part of the sweetener in it. Instead, give less at first and add later if necessary. The specific amount depends on the sweetener used, the quality and "strength" of the chocolate and, of course, your taste. So possibly adjust it to your liking.
7. Stir the gelatin into the hot cream and let it dissolve. If you use powder, add it now, without soaking it first.
8. Set aside the hot cream and stir in the cream cheese. You can also use a submersible mixer. The mass will be smoother, without lumps, but count on the formation of air bubbles in the mixture (which does not affect the taste).
9. Now comes a little math! Pour a little less than half of the cream into the cake tin on the cooled body.
10. Take 2/3 of what you have left and carefully mix less than half of the hot chocolate (the second part of the stated weight) into them. Again, you can use an immersion mixer. Ensure that the chocolate is not too cold and does not start to solidify too quickly in the mixture.

11. Pour the mixture into the center of the white cream. This will create a darker wheel in the middle of the white (do not spread or stir anything).
12. Pour the rest of the cream mixture into the pot where you have most of the melted chocolate left and mix well again. Pour the darkest cream in the middle of the light brown to create a third round (don't mix anything again).
13. Put the prepared cake in the fridge and let it cool down minimally 4 hours, ideally overnight.
14. Before serving, remove the cake from the mold, grate a few grams of dark chocolate, cut it into pieces and serve.

32. Cauliflower Croquettes

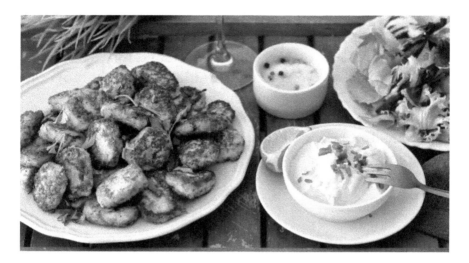

Preparation: 15 minutes
Cooking / baking: 20 minutes
Quantity: 3 servings

Ingredients:
- 600 g of cauliflower
- 90 g mayonnaise
- 1 + 2 cloves of garlic
- 100 g grated parmesan cheese
- 2 eggs
- 1 large handful of fresh parsley
- salt
- pepper
- frying fat (lard, ghee)

Method:
1. Crush cauliflower in a blender into a fine pulp. This time it doesn't have to be grains like rice, quite the opposite. The finer the crumb, the better.

92

2. Salt the cauliflower. There is no need to save salt, give a full spoon. Mix well and let stand for a while.
3. Meanwhile, prepare the garlic mayonnaise. Just mix unflavored mayonnaise with 1 clove of finely crushed garlic. Alternatively, fatty sour cream or yogurt can be used. Let the dip cool down.
4. Squeeze the crushed cauliflower carefully in a clean cotton cloth as dry as possible. It will give you work by entrusting your partner with it or taking it as a small strength training exercise. The drier the pulp, the better it will hold the croquettes together. The weight of cauliflower should be reduced by almost half.
5. Mix the squeezed cauliflower with grated parmesan cheese and eggs. Add 2 mashed cloves of garlic and finely chopped herbs. Instead of parsley, you can also use, for example, lovage, basil, onion, chives, etc. Back the mixture, taste it, and, if necessary, add a little salt.
6. Make small croquettes out of the dough. You can make balls, but small cubes are better because you can be sure that they will be toasted on all sides. Expect them to drop slightly in your pan, so make them a little higher. Approximately 50 of these amounts out at a weight of about 12 g per croquet.
7. In a pan, heat a higher layer of fat to a higher medium temperature and fry the prepared croquettes in it. Because their height in the hot fat decreases slightly, it is enough to bake them from 2 sides. From each way3 minutes.
8. Move the fried croquettes from the pan to a paper towel, which will pull out the excess fat. Allow them to cool slightly, and then serve them with a chilled garlic dip.

33. Mushroom Soup with Brie Cheese

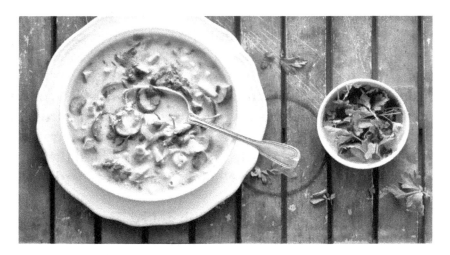

Preparation: 5 minutes
Cooking / baking: 25 minutes
Quantity: 2 servings as a main course

Ingredients:
- 50 g butter
- 75 g of onion
- 50 g of leek
- 50 g celery stalks
- 50 g carrots
- 250 g fresh mushrooms (mushrooms, champignons, oyster)
- 1 DCL of dry white wine (or 2 teaspoons of vinegar)
- 150 g of Brie cheese (or Camembert or laid-down Camembert)
- 500 ml of broth or water
- salt
- pepper
- fresh parsley

Method:
1. In a wider pot, fry the diced and lightly salted onion until pink on medium heat.
2. Add finely chopped vegetables (leeks, celery, carrots) and also fry until finely golden. Pour the chopped mushrooms over the roasted vegetables into larger pieces and let them fry, stirring occasionally.
3. Pour dry white wine over the contents of the pot and let it boil while stirring constantly. If you smell the mixture of mushrooms and vegetables, the wine should not be smelled from it.
4. Pour broth over the vegetable mixture and bring to a boil. As soon as the soup starts to boil, slightly lower the hotplate's temperature, pour the diced cheese into the pot (expect it to dissolve only partially) and leave everything to Cook for 10 minutes.
5. Take part of the soup aside, mix it smoothly and pour it back into the pot:
6. Season the finished soup with salt and pepper and serve it hot, sprinkled with fresh parsley.

34. Cauliflower Rice

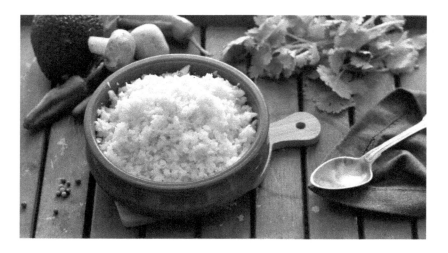

Preparation: 10 minutes
Cooking / baking: 20 minutes
Quantity: 2 servings

Ingredients:
- 600 g of cauliflower
- Salt

Method:
1. Crush cauliflower roses in a larger electric chopper (food processor) into rice-sized grains. Be sure not to use an immersion or table mixer. You need a device where the cutting edges rotate horizontally around the center axis. Don't even use small sticks for a stick mixer. Otherwise, you will have couscous from cauliflower instead of rice (but even that is sometimes useful).
2. If you do not have an electric cleaver, you can grate the cauliflower on a coarse grater or chop it finely with a knife. In both cases, however, expect to have cauliflower throughout the kitchen.

3. Heat-treat the cauliflower grains so that they soften and also lose their typical aroma. You have more options again.

4. This treatment is enough to salt (do not pour) the grains and cook them in suitable container8-12 minutes at full power, with 2-3 mixes. The exact time depends on the number of portions being prepared and the power of your microwave.

5. If you do not have a microwave oven or are avoiding using it, simmer the crushed cauliflower in a pan under the lid. Do not cover it; just salt it and simmer it covered at a low temperature with occasional stirring10-15 minutes. Then uncover the lid and leave it to still Boil in excess liquid for 5 minutes.

6. Serve cauliflower rice as you are used to with the classic one; it is suitable as a great side dish to various meat mixtures or sauces. It can be tasted as needed with various spices (such as curry or turmeric) or herbs (parsley, tarragon, coriander, oregano, etc.).

7. You can store cooked cauliflower rice in a refrigerator covered for 2-3 days, and it will last in the freezer for several months.

35. Beetroot Brownie Cake

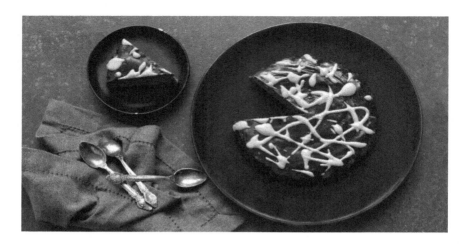

Preparation: 1 hour
Cooking/baking: 40 minutes
Quantity: 6 servings

Ingredients:
- 200 g peeled boiled beets
- 50 g sweetener (honey, coconut sugar, date syrup, erythritol, xylitol, etc. - choose a specific type and amount according to your nutritional style)
- 3 eggs
- 30 + 20 g of ghee or butter
- 100 g almond flour
- 25 g of bitter cocoa
- 8 g of baking powder with tartar or 5 g of ordinary
- 30 g of dark high percentage chocolate
- 25 g of coconut butter
- coconut milk (a couple of spoons as needed)

Method:
1. Mix the pre-cooked beetroot (available at Lidl) with the sweetener of your choice. Set aside one teaspoon of the mixture, add eggs and 30 g of softened ghee to the rest.
2. Next, mix almond flour, cocoa and baking powder.
3. Mix the two mixtures and pour the dough into a cake tin (I used a diameter of 17 cm), lined with baking paper, which you first crumpled and moistened for easier handling.
4. Put the dough in an oven heated to 180 ° C and bake for approximately 40 minutes. The exact time can vary greatly depending on the height of the dough.
5. To find out if the body is already baked, insert a stick into its center and check that it comes out clean. If so, you're done.
6. Remove the body from the oven and let it cool down. Once it is at room temperature, put it in the fridge or the freezer for a few minutes. We need its surface to be very cold.
7. In a small pan, heat 20 g of butter and dark chocolate to a low temperature. Allow the mixture to cool for a while, and then spread the cold cake with it from the top and sides with a masher. Thanks to its cooling, the chocolate on its surface will solidify faster.
8. Heat the coconut butter in the microwave in a small cup. Then, carefully, in small portions, mix in the mixed beets you have set aside. The mixture thickens relatively, so gently dilute it with a little coconut milk as needed and the desired color. Drizzle the cake with this mixture and let it cool for a while.
9. Then just enjoy it

36. Homemade Cini Minis

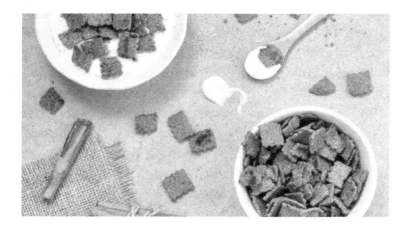

Preparation: 5 minutes
Cooking / baking: 30 minutes
Amount: 4 servings

Ingredients:
- 50 g almond flour
- 15 g of coconut flour
- 30 g of coconut oil, ghee, or butter
- 1 protein
- 1 teaspoon ground cinnamon
- approximately. 25 g of sweetener (honey, coconut sugar, date syrup, erythritol, xylitol, etc. - choose a specific type and amount according to your nutritional style)

Method:
1. Prepare all the listed ingredients into a medium-firm dough. If you use dates, chop them into as small pieces as possible.
2. Roll the dough between two baking papers into a thin pancake (1-2 mm). Carefully peel off the top paper and cut the sheet into small cubes (approximately 1 x 1 cm).

3. Place the prepared squares in an oven preheated to 150 ° C and bake for approximately 15 minutes with the mixer inserted in the oven door (so that it does not close and moisture can escape from the oven). Then switch off the oven and let the cini minis run in it.
4. Serve the finished cinnamon squares as you are used to, for example, with yogurt or milk; it is also great as a small snack or a travel treat.
5. Store in a closed container, where the cini minis will last for several weeks.

37. "Semolina" Cashew Porridge

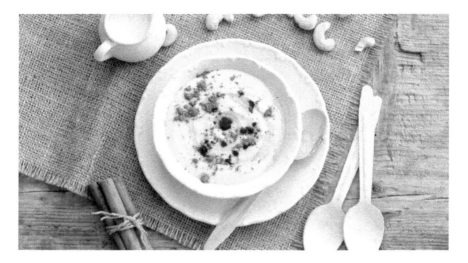

Preparation: 2 hours
Cooking / baking: 5 minutes
Quantity: 2 servings

Ingredients:
- 80 g cashew nuts (unsalted, unroasted)
- 350 ml of coconut or classic milk, or diluted cream *
- sweetener according to your eating style and taste (honey, dates, date syrup, xylitol, erythritol, etc.)
- 2 teaspoons ghee or butter
- ground cinnamon or bitter cocoa

Method:
1. To make cashew nuts as digestible as possible, soak them at least for 2 hours (or overnight if you are preparing porridge for breakfast) in water with a pinch of salt added. But you can skip this step altogether. Sometimes it's a hurry, I understand, but you need a really powerful mixer that can mix cashew nuts well.

2. Just before preparing the porridge, drain the nuts, rinse them with fresh water, and dry.
3. Mix the dripped nuts smoothly with coconut milk. Let it matter. We don't want any lumps in the porridge, so give it time.
4. Once the mixture is beautifully smooth, pour it into a small pan and bring to a boil, constantly stirring, to a medium temperature. The mixture must be bubbling. As soon as it goes through the boiling, the porridge thickens beautifully. And a little more to partially cool during serving.
5. Taste the finished "semolina" porridge and sweeten it if necessary. But mostly, it is not necessary; cashews and coconut milk are naturally sweet in themselves.
6. Serve the porridge warm, drizzled with melted ghee or butter, and sprinkled with cinnamon or cocoa.

38. Home Lučina

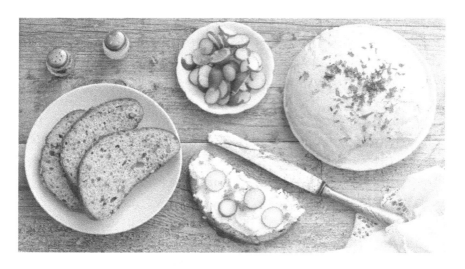

Preparation: 8 hours
Quantity: 4 servings

Ingredients:
- 400 g of fatty yogurt (preferably Greek or rustic)
- 150 g whipping cream min. 30%
- salt
- herbs, sun-dried tomatoes, nuts, spices, etc. to taste

Method:
1. Whisk the cream and then work it very gently into the yogurt.
2. Depending on your taste, mix in a little salt and possibly other ingredients such as chopped herbs or nuts, finely chopped dried tomatoes, or your favorite spices (such as sweet pepper or turmeric). Of course, you can also leave the cheese completely clean, without flavor, only with salt.
3. Pour the mixture into a sufficiently large sieve or colander lined with a clean cotton cloth or several gauze layers.

4. Place a small plate on top, which has a smaller diameter than the colander, so that it will lie on the surface of the mixture with its entire surface and weigh it slightly with its weight.
5. Place the sieve on a pot or bowl deep enough so that the strainer's bottom is not too low and does not bathe later in the drained liquid.
6. Put the pot with the colander in the fridge and leave the mixture there for at least 8 hours to drip.
7. After dripping, carefully tip the contents of the sieve onto a plate and remove the gauze or cloth from the surface of the pile.
8. Done! You have your own beautifully fluffy Lučina ready. You can use it classically to spread popular pastries (such as yogurt or seed bread) or prepare other dishes (salmon roulade, etc.).
9. The finished cheese will stay covered in the fridge for several days.

39. Cold Tomato Soup Salmorejo

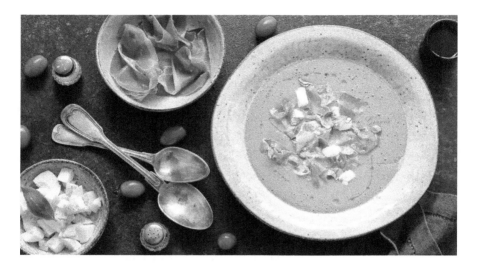

Preparation: 15 minutes
Cooking / baking: 10 minutes
Quantity: 2 servings

Ingredients:
- 500 g ripe tomatoes *
- 2 larger cloves of garlic
- 1 tablespoon wine or balsamic vinegar
- 20 g shallots
- 50 g of sunflower butter or hazelnut
- 1 DCL of cold water
- salt
- pepper
- 3 eggs
- 50 g quality dried ham (does not apply to the vegetarian variant)
- 1 tablespoon olive oil

Method:
1. If you have small tomatoes (such as cherry or date palm), use them whole.
2. I recommend peeling them first for large tomatoes - cut the skin crosswise, boil the tomatoes in boiling water, and then cool rapidly in ice. The skin is easy to peel off. In addition to peeling, cut large tomatoes and dig out the watery center with a spoon's seeds. Throw him out.
3. Mix the prepared tomatoes with peeled garlic, diced shallots, sunflower butter, vinegar, 1 dcl of water, salt, and a little pepper.
4. Let the soup cool in the fridge. Boil the eggs hard while cooling.
5. Peel a boiled egg and cut it into cubes.
6. Serve the soup cold, sprinkled with eggs, torn slices of dried ham, and drizzled with olive oil.

40. Celery Salad

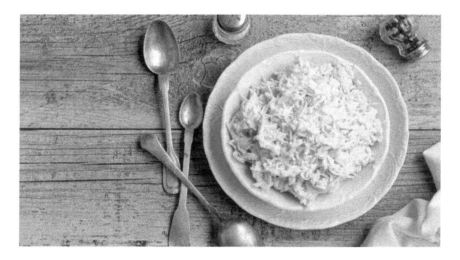

Preparation: 25 minutes
Cooking / baking: 5 minutes
Quantity: 5 servings

Ingredients:
- 500 g of celery
- 100 g carrots
- 50 g of onion
- 100 g apples (ideally some more acidic varieties)
- 200 g mayonnaise (ideally homemade)
- lemon juice as needed
- salt
- pepper

Method:
1. Finely grate the peeled celery and carrots. If you have an electric grinder or blender with an attachment, definitely use it. This will significantly reduce the preparation of vegetables.

2. Cut the onion as finely as possible. Discard the washed unpeeled apple and cut it into small cubes.
3. Bring more salted water to a boil in a large pot. In it then approximately Cook grated celery for 5 minutes.
4. Finally, drain it as much as possible and let it cool down.
5. Mix cold boiled celery with grated carrots, chopped onions, and apples.
6. Combine everything with mayonnaise and salt and pepper to your liking. Add lemon juice as needed.
7. Allow to cool.
8. Serve the celery salad as a side dish to meatballs, cutlets, or roast meat.
9. But it will also be great as a quick snack or a fresh breakfast supplement; it tastes wonderful as a non-traditional spread.
10. Stored in the refrigerator will last for several days.

TIPS:
Do not pour the celery broth over the celery. You can use it with other celery to make a soup, such as blue cheese and nuts.

It can be dripped with a little lemon to prevent the celery from turning too yellow during cooling.

If you do not avoid dairy products, you can partially replace mayonnaise with yogurt or sour cream.

41. Zucchini Poppies

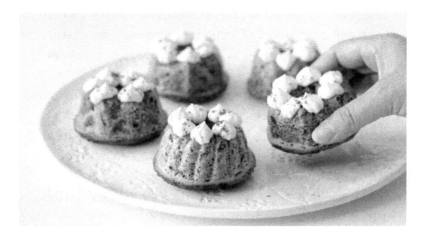

Preparation: 1 hour
Cooking / baking: 30 minutes
Quantity: 6 servings

Ingredients:
1) DOUGH
- 200 g peeled zucchini
- 2 eggs
- 100 g almond flour
- 75 g ground poppy
- approximately. 40 g sweetener (honey, coconut sugar, date syrup, erythritol, xylitol, etc. - choose a specific type and amount according to your nutritional style)
- 2 teaspoons baking powder with tartar or 1 teaspoon plain

2) CREAM
- 40 g of cream cheese (Philadelphia, Goldessa Cheese, etc.)
- 40 g butter
- approximately. 10 g sweetener (honey, coconut sugar, date syrup, erythritol, xylitol, etc. - choose a specific type and amount according to your nutritional style)

- a few drops of vanilla extract or granules of half a pod

Method:
1. Take the butter out of the fridge and let it loosen. Do not use a microwave or hotplate. We need the butter to soften but not warm.
2. Cut the peeled zucchini into cubes and mix them smoothly with eggs and the chosen sweetener. Take your time; give it time to fluff as much as possible.
3. Mix almond flour, ground poppy seeds, and tartar.
4. Add the loose ingredients to the zucchini mixture and gently work by hand into a thin dough. Do not use a blender to avoid ruining the zucchini mixture.
5. Fill the molds into mini cakes or muffins with the prepared dough and let them bake for 25-30 minutes in an oven preheated to 180 ° C.
6. While the cakes are being baked, prepare the cream. Carefully mix the softened butter with the cream cheese, selected sweetener, and vanilla. Mix everything into a perfectly smooth cream. Then put it in the refrigerator to cool down.
7. Take the baked cakes out of the oven, let them cool for a while, and then take them out of the molds.
8. Once the muffins are at room temperature, decorate them with chilled cream and serve.

42. Yogurt Pastry

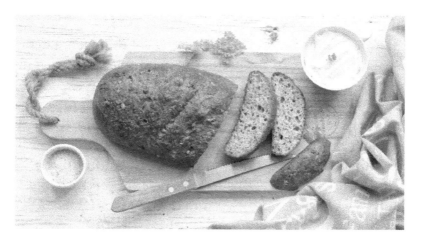

Preparation: 10 minutes
Cooking / baking: 50 minutes
Quantity: 4 servings

Ingredients:
- 150 g fatty yogurt (Greek or cream with 10% fat)
- 4 eggs M
- 5 g of salt (1 level teaspoon)
- 80 g golden flax seeds (5 full spoons)
- 20 g psyllium (2 heaped spoons)
- 50 g of a mixture of popular seeds and nuts (e.g., pumpkin, sunflower, pecans)
- 5 g of baking powder with tartar or 3 g of ordinary

Method:
1. Knock eggs into a bowl, add yogurt and salt. Mix everything thoroughly - using an immersion mixer or even a fork.
2. Finely grind flax seeds and psyllium. An electric coffee grinder or a powerful chisel will do this job very well.

3. If you want to mix nuts into the dough, crush them into smaller pieces. Ideally, put them in a bag and break them with a few strokes with a meat mallet. You would chop them too finely in a grinder or chopper. If you are adding seeds, you can leave them whole. It is not necessary to break them.

4. Mix thoroughly ground flax and psyllium, baking powder, and seeds or nuts. Add the egg mixture, really GOOD, and mix thoroughly. Leave at least Stand the dough for 2 minutes and thicken.

5. Make 2 higher loaves from the sticky medium-thick dough. The dough must not spill over the baking sheet (line it with baking paper), but it must keep its shape. If it is too liquid, it is better to incorporate a little more psyllium into it.

6. Put the loaves in an oven preheated to 160 ° C and bake approximately 50-55 minutes. Do not open the oven during this time so that the dough does not fall out unnecessarily.

7. After the set time, take out the bread, place it on a cotton or paper towel (these will help remove excess moisture from the pastry), and let it cool down. Only then can you slice the bread. If you skipped this step, the pastry would be too moist and greasy.

TIP:
If you happen to gain a lot of bread in the oven and later "collapse," use less baking powder next time.

43. Baked Walnut Sticks

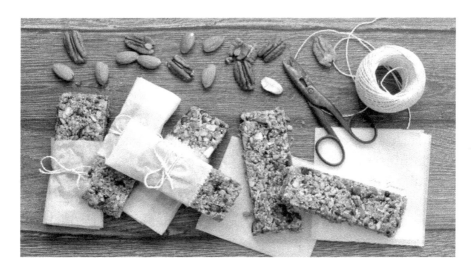

Preparation: 10 minutes
Cooking / baking: 30 minutes
Quantity: 8 bars

Ingredients:
- 20 g chia seeds (2 level spoons)
- 1 egg
- 1 protein
- 1 tablespoon lemon juice
- 30 g sweetener (honey, coconut sugar, date syrup, erythritol, xylitol, etc. - choose a specific type and amount according to your nutritional style)
- 100 g almonds (3 handfuls)
- 100 g pecans (3 handfuls)
- 20 g grated coconut (2 full tablespoons)
- 50 g sunflower seeds (3 full spoons)
- 50 g pumpkin seeds (3 full spoons)
- 20 g unsweetened dried fruit (cranberries, plums, etc.) - optional

Method:

1. Mix chia seeds with egg, egg white, sweetener, and lemon juice. Leave at least Swell for 10 minutes.
2. Roughly crush all nuts and seeds (except the chia you have already used) in a few pulses. Pour a large part of the nut-seed pulp into a bowl and mix the small residue finely with sliced dried fruit (or without, if you omit dried fruit).
3. Mix soaked chia seeds and both walnut crumbs together. Work well.
4. Line a suitable container (I used a baking dish 14 x 22 cm) with baking paper and stuff the prepared mixture well on it.
5. Place in an oven heated to 160 ° C and bake for approximately 30 minutes.
6. Cut the baked walnut plate into the required shapes and store it in a closed box in a dry place, where it will last for two weeks.

44. Milk Slices

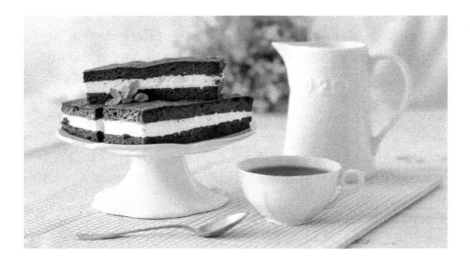

Preparation: 40 minutes
Cooking / baking: 15 minutes
Quantity: 6 slices

Ingredients:
1) DOUGH
- 4 eggs
- 100 g of cream cheese (Philadelphia, Goldessa Cheese, etc.)
- about 30 g of sweetener according to your eating style (honey, dates, date syrup, xylitol, erythritol, etc.) *
- 40 g of bitter cocoa (the exact amount depends on the type used - see TIPS)
- a pinch of salt

2) CREAM
- 250 g mascarpone
- approximately. 20 g of sweetener according to your eating style *

Method:
1. First, carefully separate the yolks from the egg whites. Because we will make snow from the proteins, you must not get even a little yolk into them. Also, be careful that the bowl in which you knock the whites and prepare snow in it is not greasy. Then you wouldn't do very well in the snow.
2. Mix the egg yolks carefully with the cream cheese and sweetener. If you use dates, cut them into smaller pieces beforehand and then mix them smoothly together with the yolks and cream cheese.
3. Gradually mix in the cocoa and work in a smooth dough. In the beginning, give it less, taste it and sprinkle it if necessary (see TIPS).
4. Beat the egg whites with a small pinch of salt into the hard snow and then work it very gently (to not destroy the bubbles in it, so do not use a mixer) into the cocoa mixture.
5. Pour the dough onto a baking sheet lined with baking paper and spread it on a rectangle approximately 1 cm high (not over the entire baking sheet, so that the pancake is not too low).
6. Place the prepared dough in a preheated oven at 160 ° C and bake 15 minutes. Do not use hot air; rather, choose lower and upper heating.
7. Take the baked body out of the oven and let it cool down. Then turn it over with the paper and carefully peel it from the dough.
8. Before the dough bakes, mix the mascarpone (be careful, it should not be too liquid; otherwise, the cream will not stick to you) with the chosen sweetener. Again, if you use dates, cut them into smaller pieces and mix them with mascarpone. Allow the prepared cream to cool in the refrigerator.

9. Cut the cooled body in half. Coat one part with chilled mascarpone and cover with the other half.
10. Cut the "cake" into 6 equal pieces, into rectangles or squares. I'll leave that to you
11. Store milk slices in the refrigerator (they will stay covered for 3 days) and serve chilled.

TIPS:
Beware of cocoa used. Some species are very pronounced and bitter, so add it gradually. I recommend not using Dutch cocoa and preferring to choose cocoa powder from unroasted beans or natural cocoa.

For example, because erythritol or xylitol sweeten less and honey, on the other hand, sweeten more, and everyone tastes an otherwise distinct sweetness, adapt the specific amount of sweetener used to your taste and eating style. Use it less, taste it and add it if necessary. Nutritional values are calculated for the use of erythritol with zero caloric value or with the omission of sweetener altogether.

Instead of cuts, a roll can also be prepared. Just spread the filling over the uncut sheet of dough and roll.

45. Zucchini Rollatini

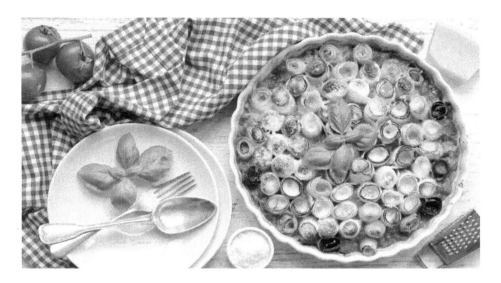

Preparation: 45 minutes
Cooking/baking: 1 hour 15 minutes
Quantity: 3 servings

Ingredients:
- 600 g zucchini (2 medium)
- 2 tablespoons olive oil
- 4 cloves garlic
- 400 g peeled tomatoes (1 can)
- 2 handfuls of fresh basil
- 300 g of ricotta or cottage cheese
- 125 g mozzarella (1 bun)
- 75 g of parmesan cheese
- salt
- pepper

Method:

1. Wash the zucchini and grate them into wider slices using a wide scraper. Whenever you get to the watery center, turn the zucchini and peel it again from the other side.

2. Cut the inner blocks left over from the zucchini into small cubes.

3. Mix the grated zucchini slices with 1/2 teaspoon of salt and let them sweat and soften on a sieve.

4. In a larger pan, heat the olive oil and fry the zucchini cubes gently on a medium temperature with a little salt and pepper. Once most of the liquid released by the vegetables has boiled, add the crushed garlic to the pan and let it rind while stirring. Pour the peeled tomatoes over the pan, sprinkle with finely chopped basil and let everything else Cook for 15 minutes. Occasionally mix the mixture and mash the tomatoes into smaller pieces.

5. Pour the finished sauce on the baking dish's bottom (I used a cake mold with a diameter of 24 cm).

6. Mix ricotta, grated mozzarella, and 50 g of grated parmesan (leave the rest for final baking). If you have an electric chopper at your disposal, you can simplify your work - first crush parmesan cubes to dust, pour 25 g aside and mix the rest with mozzarella and ricotta.

7. Gently squeeze the salted zucchini slices and dry them in a cotton cloth.

8. And now comes the most challenging part of the whole recipe. I won't lie to you; it's a pipette, but you can do it, and the result is worth it. Ideally, get a helper. Maybe kids could enjoy it.

9. Gently spread each slice of zucchini to one-third with a cheese mixture (approximately 1 teaspoon) and then roll into a roll on this side. Place the rolls on the prepared tomato sauce in a baking dish and gradually fill the whole bottom with them.

10. When all the rolls are ready, and the baking dish is full, place it in an oven heated to 190 ° C and bake 35 minutes. Then sprinkle the "cake" with 25 g of grated parmesan cheese and leave to Bake for 10 minutes.
11. Drizzle the finished zucchini rolls with olive oil, garnish with fresh basil leaves and serve while still warm. But they also taste great cold.

46. Tiramisu

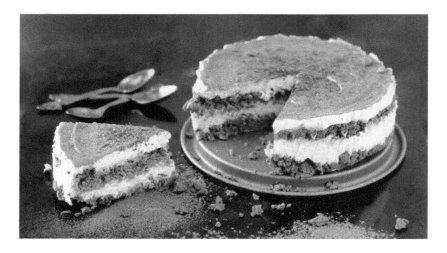

Preparation: 4 hours 30 minutes
Cooking / baking: 20 minutes
Quantity: 6 servings

Ingredients:
1) CORPUS
- 200 g of nuts or walnut butter (pecans, walnuts, hazelnuts, etc.)
- 3 eggs L or 4 eggs M
- 3 teaspoons of finely ground coffee (can be replaced with cocoa for children)
- 1 cup of baking powder with tartar or 1 teaspoon of ordinary
- 2 tablespoons rum (may be omitted)

2) CREAM
- 60 g sweetener (honey, coconut sugar, date syrup, erythritol, xylitol, etc. - choose a specific type and amount according to your nutritional style)
- 2 eggs

- a pinch of salt
- 400 g mascarpone
- 2 teaspoons of bitter cocoa

Method:
1. Crush the nuts in a suitable paste mixer to a paste or use hazelnut butter directly. Mix them with 3 or 4 eggs (depending on size), tartar, and finely ground coffee. If you only have coarser coffee, you should grind it separately so that it does not crunch between your teeth.
2. Pour the finished dough onto a baking sheet lined with baking paper and spread on a pancake 2-3 cm high. Put it in an oven heated to 150 ° C and bake for about20 minutes. The dough rises a lot during baking, and its surface cracks slightly.
3. Allow the finished body to cool (important condition), and then gently break it into small pieces between your fingers.
4. Whip the selected sweetener with 2 egg yolks. Once it dissolves, stir in the mascarpone.
5. Make hard snow from the proteins. Then mix it carefully and in portions into the yolk mixture. Work gently so that the snow does not fall and the cream does not lose its fluff.
6. Prepare a suitable container. You can also use separate bowls or glasses, a glass bowl, or a cake tin. Make a layer of the finely crushed body on the bottom, drizzle with rum, and stuff well. The next layer will be mascarpone with eggs, then a crushed body drizzled with rum and gently stuffed, then mascarpone.
7. The last layer should be a cream, which is sprinkled through the sieve with bitter cocoa.
8. Leave the tiramisu in the fridge overnight (minimum 4 hours) and then just cheer

47. Flour-Free Pasta

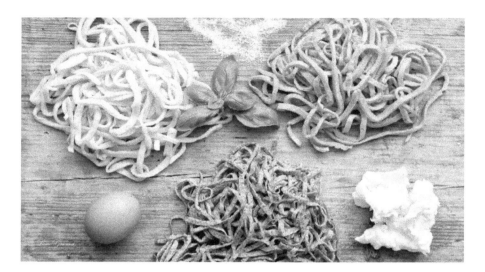

Preparation: 5 minutes
Cooking / baking: 10 minutes
Quantity: 2 servings

Ingredients:
- 5 eggs
- 1 bun of mozzarella from brine (125 g)
- 15 g psyllium (2 heaped spoons)
- salt

Method:
1. In a blender or with the help of that dipper, make eggs, mozzarella (without brine, torn to pieces), psyllium, and salt into a smooth, thin dough. The smoother the dough, the finer the pasta will be, so really care. That is why I recommend finely grinding psyllium beforehand.
2. Pour the prepared dough onto 2 sheets lined with baking paper and spread it on the thinnest possible pancakes.

Expect the dough to rise slightly, so don't be afraid to make the pancakes thin. Work fast. Baking paper easily absorbs moisture and begins to crumple. However, this can be largely prevented by gently greasing the sheet metal. The baking paper will then be added to it, and the dough will spread better.

3. Place the dough sheets in an oven preheated to 160 ° C and bake 6-8 minutes. The result should be flexible, non-dried sheets but not too wet to prevent the pasta from sticking.

4. Take the baked pancakes out of the oven and turn them over with the paper. Then gently peel it off.

5. Roll the still warm pancakes into a roll and use a sharp knife to cut them into thin strips.

6. Serve the finished pasta as usual - for example, with tomato sauce, pesto, parmesan, "aglio olio e peperoncino" or as a supplement to Asian dishes, etc. You can cut them into thicker fettuccine-style noodles, or even leave them whole and use them as lasagna.

7. Baked pasta can be stored covered in the refrigerator for several days, in the freezer for several months. Just use them briefly in a pan or microwave before use.

8. If you want to play with colors and flavors, you can mix different ingredients into the dough, such as spinach, sun-dried tomatoes, basil, turmeric, pepper, chili, etc. But always choose one that will fit into the final dish.

48. Cauliflower "Gnocchi"

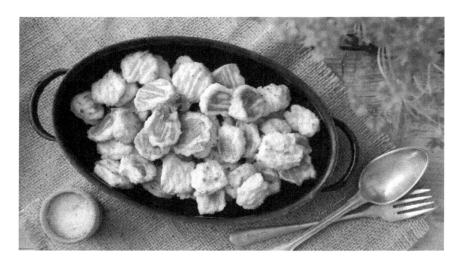

Preparation: 15 minutes
Cooking / baking: 40 minutes
Quantity: 3 servings

Ingredients:
- 700 g cauliflower (1 small)
- 240 g mozzarella (2 pieces)
- 4 egg yolks
- salt
- pepper

Method:
1. First, prepare the cauliflower. You have more options, but the result should be a soft and as dry matter as possible.
2. One of the variants is to boil cauliflower roses gently in saltwater. Pour them and then squeeze in a clean cotton cloth. It's a bit of a gym but squeeze until even a drop of fluid flows. We need the pulp as dry as possible.

3. Another option is to cook cauliflower in a microwave oven. Cut it into small pieces or crush in a blender, then "ripple" the salted ones with occasional mixing for about10 minutes (exact time depends on your oven's performance). Then, as in the previous case, squeeze the cooked cauliflower perfectly with a cotton cloth.
4. In both cases, let the cauliflower soften a lot. Not only will the resulting dough be softer, but most of the typical, unpleasant, typical cauliflower flavors and aromas will disappear.
5. Another ingredient is mozzarella. Here, too, we need to get rid of excess moisture. Tear it into pieces and then dissolve them either in a microwave oven or at a lower temperature in a small saucepan on a hot plate. It should soften and separate the cream. Drain it and use it for another recipe or to soften the sauce for cauliflower "gnocchi."
6. In a blender, process squeezed cauliflower and fused mozzarella into a smooth, medium-thin dough (let both ingredients cool down a little), egg yolks, salt, and pepper. Make tiny buns out of the mass and place them on a baking sheet lined with baking paper. If you have squeezed cauliflower and mozzarella well, the dough should have exactly the right consistency so that it sticks a little to your fingers, but you can work with it and with the help of a fork, you could print typical grooves on the buns.
7. Place the prepared baking dish with "gnocchi" in an oven heated to 180 ° C and bake for approximately 20 minutes until golden.
8. Serve the finished "gnocchi" as usual. They taste great with creamy mushroom sauce, roasted bacon and asparagus, sun-dried tomatoes and herb pesto, and many other combinations.

49. Chocolate Fondant

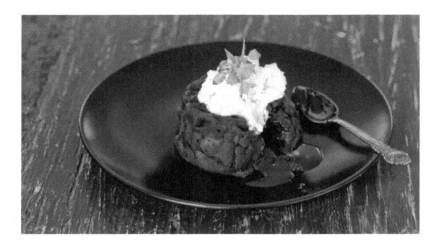

Preparation: 10 minutes
Cooking / baking: 10 minutes
Quantity: 2 servings

Ingredients:
- 50 g of dark high percentage chocolate (min. 85%)
- 60 g butter
- 2 eggs
- 5 g of bitter cocoa
- 15 g sweetener (honey, coconut sugar, date syrup, erythritol, xylitol, etc. - choose a specific type and amount according to your nutritional style)
- 20 g walnut butter (almonds, cashews, etc.)

Method:
1. Switch on the oven at 220 ° C and let it heat up.
2. Melt the butter in the microwave or on a hot plate. Remove one tablespoon, melt the rest of the chocolate and mix into a smooth mixture.

3. In another bowl, beat the eggs with the sweetener. You can omit this altogether. It depends on your taste and also on the sugar content of the chocolate used. Of course, the less, the better.
4. Stir nut butter and a pinch of bitter cocoa in a tablespoon of melted butter that you have set aside. You should get a thin brown mixture. We will use this as the center of the fondant.
5. Mix the prepared eggs and the chocolate mixture. Work everything into a smooth, thinner dough. If you have heated the chocolate with the butter too much, let it cool down a little before connecting it to the eggs so that the eggs do not boil before putting them in the oven. To the touch, the chocolate mixture should only be lukewarm, not hot.
6. Carefully wipe the porcelain bowls (suitable for the oven) with butter (it's great with a butter wrapper) and sprinkle with a little bitter cocoa. Every piece of the bottom and the wall should be covered so that the dough does not stick to them and the fondant does not tear when tipped.
7. The bowls should not be too low so that the dough does not burn too quickly in them and you do not lose the effect with a liquid center (but we will support it with a filling of walnut butter). I have tried these from Tescom, for example.
8. Fill the prepared bowls with 2/3 of the dough, divide the walnut butter mixture on top and cover with the rest of the chocolate dough. The bowls should be 2/3 full. Expect to get a lot of dough, so do not fill the bowls to the brim.
9. Put the prepared cakes in a preheated oven and bake 8-10 minutes, depending on its performance. It worked out for me to leave the fondants in the oven exactly at home9 minutes. So, the dough is baked, but it does not dry out, and the inside remains beautifully liquid.

10. Carefully tip the still hotcakes onto the plates. If your top is torn off, it doesn't matter so much. Gently dig it out of the bowl and place it on top of the fondant.
11. Top up the chocolate cakes to taste with, for example, vanilla ice cream, whipped cream, or a spoonful of mascarpone and serve immediately. Boiled forest fruit sauce is also great.

50. Eggplant Falafel

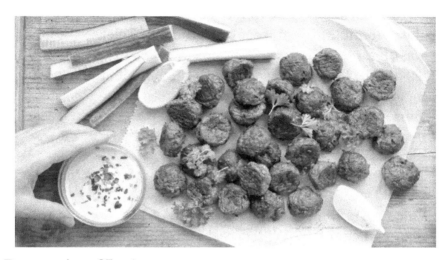

Preparation: 25 minutes
Cooking / baking: 40 minutes
Quantity: 3 servings

Ingredients:
- 300 g eggplant (1 medium)
- 2 tablespoons olive oil
- 75 g onion (1 medium)
- 10 g garlic (3 smaller cloves)
- 250 g Halloumi cheese *
- 1 egg
- 1 teaspoon sweet pepper
- 1 teaspoon crushed cumin
- 1 teaspoon dried oregano
- salt
- pepper

Method:

1. Cut the washed unpeeled eggplant into approximately centimeter slices. Spread them on a paper towel and salt them abundantly. At least leave them to Release the liquid for 10 minutes.
2. Then turn them over, salt them again and let the water run again.
3. Rinse the sweaty eggplant slices with water to remove excess salt and squeeze as much as possible. Cut into cubes.
4. Heat olive oil in a pan and let the finely chopped onion glaze over it.
5. Once the onion has softened, add the crushed garlic and chopped eggplant. With occasional stirring, leave the vegetable mixture to medium temperature until the eggplant has softened and the excess liquid has evaporated. Then set aside the pan and allow the mixture to cool.
6. In a blender, crush the chopped Halloumi cheese to the coarser sand's consistency and pour it into a bowl.
7. Then roughly mix the chilled fried eggplant with one egg. Add the mixture to a bowl of crushed cheese, sprinkle with paprika, dried oregano, and pepper. There is usually no need to add salt. Halloumi cheese is quite salty in itself; some salt remains in the eggplant.
8. Make the mixture into a thinner but moldable dough. If it is too thin, you can mix 1-2 tablespoons of almond flour into it. Make about 30 balls of the mixture on a baking sheet lined with baking paper and bake in a preheated oven at 180 ° C for15-20 minutes until they start to turn golden. Do not bake them unnecessarily so that they do not dry out.
9. Serve the finished balls as you are used to with classic falafel. You can wrap them in oopsie cakes or cut lots of

fresh vegetables and add an interesting dip. This can be flavored mayonnaise, yogurt mixed with herbs, or tahini sauce (sesame tahini diluted with water, flavored with lemon, salt, pepper, and chili, dripped with a little olive oil).

Conclusion

A high intake of grains, legumes, and starchy vegetables is involved in most vegetarian diets. Vegetarians are never absolutely complete for this purpose. Compatible for most vegetarian diets is the ketogenic diet.

However, for vegans who do not eat dairy products or eggs, the keto diet is not appropriate. It is difficult to eat enough every day without animal origin products, respecting the proportion of macronutrients.

Pescatarians would be the most advantaged because they already eat fatty fish to follow a ketogenic meal plan.

The ketogenic diet simply consists of going from one diet that forces your body to burn sugar to allow your body to burn fat, as you already know. The truth is that sugar (glucose) is often burned first by the body. The body utilizes the accumulated body fat for energy as there is no more glucose to burn.

A maximum of 20 grams of carbohydrates are eaten every day in the optimal ketogenic diet, and fats, proteins, and vegetables are favored. This means that with carbohydrate-rich foods like rice, bread, potatoes, and pasta, as well as sugars in general, you may need to make a clean break. Although the keto diet is an ideal diet plan for those trying to see their body weight actually shift, 100 percent of any diet can also be hard to adhere to.

We are all invited to birthday parties, weddings, or, from time to time, just want to enjoy a day of independence. If you are adopting a ketogenic diet, what complicates the matter is that indulging in certain sweets will bring us out of the ketosis state, which is the one in which we burn fat. All of this being said, without feeling bad for preventing ketosis, there are some tricks we can use to override it. Significant things to remember about ketosis when taking a day off

Firstly, brace yourself with snacks and with the mental knowledge, there will be temptations if you attend a case. For instance, you can opt to make your day of trouble coincide with an event like a birthday party or an office party, and you won't go wrong many times in a row in this way. You may also opt not to consume extra carbohydrates first.

Another way to limit temptation is to have a full stomach to attend the function. Sugary sweets can seem less inviting if you are loaded — plan before going out to have a satisfying ketogenic meal.

Many people argue that exogenous ketones and increased MCT oil intake will help keep you in a ketosis state. These arguments, however, are not solid enough because they are focused on measuring ketones in urine or breath that do not give precise results.

CPSIA information can be obtained
at www.ICGtesting.com
Printed in the USA
BVHW070816070521
606649BV00002B/488